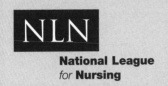

National League
for **Nursing**

TEACHING WITH ACES

ADVANCING CARE EXCELLENCE
FOR SENIORS

A FACULTY GUIDE

Edited by:

M. Elaine Tagliareni, EdD, RN, CNE, FAAN

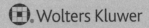. Wolters Kluwer

Philadelphia · Baltimore · New York · London
Buenos Aires · Hong Kong · Sydney · Tokyo

Executive Editor: Sherry Dickinson
Product Director: Jennifer K. Forestieri
Development Editor: Meredith L. Brittain
Production Project Manager: Cynthia Rudy
Design Coordinator: Terry Mallon
Illustration Coordinator: Jennifer Clements
Manufacturing Coordinator: Karin Duffield
Marketing Manager: Todd McQueston
Prepress Vendor: Aptara, Inc.

9 8 7 6 5 4 3 2 1

Printed in the United States of America

Library of Congress Cataloging-in-Publication Data

Names: Tagliareni, M. Elaine, editor. | National League for Nursing,
  sponsoring body.
Title: Teaching with ACE.S : a faculty guide / edited by M. Elaine Tagliareni.
Other titles: Teaching with Advancing Care Excellence for Seniors
Description: Philadelphia : Wolters Kluwer, [2017] | "National League for
  Nursing." | Includes bibliographical references.
Identifiers: LCCN 2016026711 | ISBN 9781934758274 (alk. paper)
Subjects: | MESH: Teaching–methods | Education, Nursing–methods | Geriatric
  Nursing–education
Classification: LCC RT73 | NLM WY 105 | DDC 610.73071–dc23
LC record available at https://lccn.loc.gov/2016026711

DRC0816

Andrea Mengel
1948–2016
In Memoriam

This book is dedicated to Dr. Andrea (Andy) Mengel. Andy was the heart and soul of the ACE.S project from its inception in 2007. Those of us who were fortunate to work with Andy will remember her sense of humor, attention to detail (she often said that she could edit the Gettysburg Address), and her passion for excellence in nursing education. Andy was our strongest supporter. She is greatly missed.

About the Editor

M. Elaine Tagliareni, EdD, RN, CNE, FAAN is currently a chief program officer and director of the NLN Center for Excellence in Care of Vulnerable Populations at the National League for Nursing, Washington, DC. For over 25 years, Dr. Tagliareni was a professor of nursing and the Independence Foundation Chair in Community Health Nursing Education at Community College of Philadelphia. She also served as president of the NLN from 2007 to 2009; in that position she worked to reframe the dialogue concerning entry into practice to focus on developing and supporting models that increase the academic progression of all nursing graduates, from LPN to baccalaureate to masters' and doctoral programs, to build a more diverse and educated workforce. In her role as independence foundation chair, she has served as 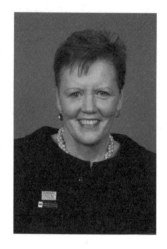 president of the National Nursing Centers Consortium (NNCC) to advance state and federal health policy to include nurse-managed health centers as essential safety net providers for older adults and other vulnerable populations.

Dr. Tagliareni has a long history of organizational leadership and grant-funded initiatives, funded through the W. K. Kellogg Foundation, the National Institute of General Medical Sciences, National Institutes of Health, The John A. Hartford Foundation, Independence Foundation and the Independence Blue Cross Foundation and to advance nursing practice and education, increase the diversity of the nursing workforce and promote educational mobility for all nurses through the creation, implementation, and dissemination of new educational models. From 2012-2015 she was the PI on a Hearst-Foundations-funded project to disseminate the NLN Advancing Care Excellence for Seniors (ACE.S) program to faculty nationally.

Dr. Tagliareni received her BSN from Georgetown University School of Nursing, a master's degree in Mental Health and Community Nursing from the University of California, San Francisco, and her doctorate from Teachers College, Columbia University.

About the Contributors

Ann P. Aschenbrenner, PhD, RN, CNE is a clinical associate professor and master of nursing program director at University of Wisconsin: Milwaukee, College of Nursing. Dr. Aschenbrenner has a long history of clinical practice and research in the areas of pediatric nursing and end-of-life care. She received her BSN from the University of Wisconsin-Milwaukee and her MSN and PhD from Marquette University, Milwaukee.

Linda M. Blazovich, DNP, RN, CNE is an associate professor of nursing at St. Catherine University and is the director of simulation in the nursing program. She introduced simulation to the nursing program in 2006 and has been instrumental in the integration of simulation into all levels of the nursing curriculum. Dr. Blazovich was trained in simulation theory and techniques at the Mayo Simulation Center in Rochester, MN and is skilled in scenario development, simulation facilitation, and debriefing. She has done research, co-authored articles, and presented at national and international conferences on simulation.

Michele Cislo, MA, RN is an associate professor of practical nursing at Union County College in Plainfield, New Jersey. She is a 2012 recipient of the New Jersey League of Nursing Nurse Recognition Award and the 2014 recipient of the NLN Hearst Foundation Excellence in Geriatric Education Award. She received a Bachelor's of Science in Nursing from William Paterson University and a Master's Degree in Nursing Education from New York University.

Daniel D. Cline, PhD, RN is an assistant professor at Samuel Merritt University School of Nursing in Oakland, California. Dr. Cline is a 2010–2012 Building Academic Geriatric Nursing Capacity (BAGNC) Predoctoral Scholar and former National League for Nursing ACE.S program manager. He currently teaches medical-surgical nursing, gerontological nursing, and health assessment in the pre-licensure BSN program at Samuel Merritt University and his research/scholarly interests include geriatrics, quality of care, systems science, and rural health.

JoAnn G. Crownover, DNP, RN, CNE is an associate professor for Loretto Heights School of Nursing (LHSON), Regis University. Prior to her employment with Regis University, Dr. Crownover taught in various academic settings, including Colorado State University-Pueblo, Adams State University, Trinidad State Junior College and Northland Pioneer College.

Dr. Crownover's specific interest in education is in innovative instructional pedagogy. She has extensive experience in the development and implementation of Nursing Simulation. She was selected as one of the 20 nurse educators from across the United States to be involved with the Inaugural National League for Nursing's Leadership Development Program for Simulation Educators. Since 2011, Dr. Crownover has been working with Dr. Kerry Reid Searl from CQ University, Australia, in the implementation of Mask-Ed, a unique and innovative simulation technique.

Dr. Crownover received her BSN from Loretto Heights College (1982), her MSN from Northern Arizona University (1997), and her DNP from Regis University (2012). She received her certification as a Nurse Educator (CNE) and is a recognized National Leader in Nursing Simulation from the National League of Nursing (NLN).

Tamika Curry, MSN, RN is an assistant professor in the Department of Nursing at Community College of Philadelphia. She is actively involved with the 19130 Zip Code Project at the College, a service-learning program to provide direct client services to at-risk and underserved clients in the 19130 zip code of Philadelphia and other surrounding areas. As a lead faculty in the NLN Advancing Care Excellence for Seniors (ACE.S) project, Ms. Curry helped to develop the ACE.S framework and has participated in the dissemination of ACE.S, providing faculty development workshops and webinars throughout the U.S. Her current research interests include: Social Determinants of Health, Health Disparities in Minority Populations, Equity in Higher Education, and College Success of Urban Students. She is currently a PhD student at Temple University in the College of Education, within the Urban Education department.

Laurie Dorsey, MSN, RN is a professor of nursing and the director of simulation at Ivy Tech Community College in Madison, IN. Ms. Dorsey also teaches for Indiana University East and Indiana Wesleyan University in the Bachelor of Science in Nursing Programs. She was in the inaugural class of the NLN Simulation Leadership Program and is a strong advocate of the value of simulation as clinical experience for nursing students.

Susan G. Forneris, PhD, RN, CNE, CHSE-A is the excelsior deputy director, Center for Innovation in Simulation and Technology, National League for Nursing, Washington, DC. Selected for inclusion in the 2010 inaugural group of NLN Simulation Leaders, she has been working in the field of clinical simulation since 2007. Dr. Forneris' expertise is in curriculum development with emphasis on simulation and debriefing in combination with her research on critical thinking. She served as a simulation expert for the NLN ACE.S team (Advancing Care Excellence for Seniors) and a simulation author for the NLN ACE.Z Alzheimer's Simulation Scenario series. Dr. Forneris is actively engaged in initiating multisite simulation research on simulation and debriefing and in the area of high-stakes testing with the MN Consortium for Nursing Education and Research. She has several publications focused on the development and use of reflective teaching strategies. Formerly, she was a professor of nursing at St. Catherine University, St. Paul, MN.

Vivienne Friday, EdD, RN has been a professional nurse for more than 36 years, with almost 10 years in academia. She is currently an associate director at the Bridgeport Hospital School of Nursing and teaches Community Health Nursing in the online RN to BSN program at the University of Bridgeport. Her practice areas included hotels, schools, hospitals, nursing homes, and academic settings. Dr. Friday is passionate about geriatric nursing. As an educator, she is committed to advancing the science of aging by maintaining a research focus on geriatric nursing, and has provided leadership in the development of geriatric courses and teaching strategies, supported by ACE.S resources. She has authored and received grants to support service learning projects in long-term care facilities and is a recipient of the 2013 NLN Hearst Foundations Excellence in Geriatric Education Award.

Walter Groteluschen, MS is an adjunct faculty member at Minnesota State University, Mankato teaching a junior/senior level statistics course. He consults on research projects for dissertations, conference presentations, and publications. He assists with designing the study, processing the data, interpreting the results, and verifying the accuracy of the written explanations. He checks for consistency and verifies that values from the data analysis have been correctly entered in the document.

Ann E. Holland, PhD, RN is a professor of nursing at Bethel University in St. Paul, MN. She practiced for 17 years in staff nurse, education, and leadership roles in critical-care nursing. Her academic experience includes six years of administration in higher education. Dr. Holland teaches nursing fundamentals, medical/surgical nursing, leadership, and health policy. She has conducted research in topics ranging from the teaching of race and racism in nursing, simulation debriefing, and innovations in clinical education. She is currently the principal investigator of a study investigating the effect of a training intervention on the reliability of evaluator ratings of student performance in clinical simulation.

Eunice S. King, PhD, RN served as senior program officer and director of research and evaluation for the Independence Foundation from 2000 until her retirement in 2015. During that time, she oversaw the foundation's grant making under the nurse-managed health care initiative and provided program evaluation consultation and technical support for many of the foundation's grantee programs, including the ACE.S project. Upon completion of her PhD studies in 1988, Dr. King joined the behavioral research staff of the Fox Chase Cancer Center Division of Population Science, where she conducted and evaluated health education programs, and later served as associate dean for research in the MCP Hahnemann School of Nursing (now Drexel University), where she taught graduate research courses.

Judith A. Kopka, MSN, RN, CNE is a clinical instructor at the University of Wisconsin: Milwaukee, College of Nursing. Ms. Kopka has many years' experience in psychiatric and geropsychiatric nursing. Her teaching experience includes mental health, gerontology, community health, end of life, and clinical simulation. She was a FLAG Fellow through the University of Minnesota Hartford Center for Geriatric Nursing Excellence and a member of the Midwest Geriatric Nursing Alliance. Affiliations during article preparation were UW: Milwaukee (as described above) and Columbia College of Nursing, Glendale, Wisconsin.

Kelly Krumwiede, PhD, RN, PHN is a nurse educator with Minnesota State University, Mankato. Dr. Krumwiede teaches community and public health nursing in the basic nursing program and is the basic nursing program coordinator. Scientific interests include development of simulation scenarios that teach how to provide care to populations with the emphasis of care of families, health promotion, and improving societal health outcomes. Dr. Krumwiede has been published in peer-reviewed journals including *Public Health Nursing Journal* and *Oncology Forum*. Her professional service includes the Glen Taylor Nursing Institute for Family and Society and Henry Street Consortium.

Norma Krumwiede, EdD, MEd, MN, RN is employed by Minnesota State University, Mankato as a nursing professor. In 2013, Dr. Krumwiede and her colleagues were awarded the Hearst Foundations' Excellence in Geriatric Education Award for their work with the National League for Nursing (NLN) ACE.S Unfolding Cases. She has published in several peer-reviewed journals including *Clinical Simulation in Nursing*, *Journal of Nursing Education*, and *Journal of Family Nursing*, and she is co-editor of a book titled: *Family Focused Care: Think Family and Transform Nursing Practice* (F. A. Davis, 2016). Since 1994, Dr. Krumwiede has taught in the undergraduate and graduate nursing programs, where she has assisted in creating "The Modern Nursing Lab," which offers a full range of simulation experiences. She also continues to research the effectiveness of simulated teaching and learning, consults with undergraduate nursing programs throughout the country, mentors new faculty with teaching and scholarship, and continues to advance the science and art of simulation through research, education, and practice.

Mary Beth Kuehn, EdD, RN, PHN is currently an assistant professor of nursing at St. Olaf College. Dr. Kuehn has been a nurse educator for the past 24 years. She has served as a CCNE site visitor for pre-licensure accreditation. Her publications focus on the lived experience of nursing faculty in the academic workplace, adolescent nonmedical prescription drug use and parental consent, and enhancing clinical reasoning through simulation debriefing. Dr. Kuehn is a member of the Minnesota Consortium for Nursing Education Research (MCNER) focused on simulation and debriefing, specifically clinical reasoning with baccalaureate nursing students. This team received the 2012 Debra L. Spunt minigrant for simulation research and the 2013 Sigma Theta Tau International—Chi Chapter at large professional development grant to promote scholarship among members. In collaboration with Dr. Diana Neal, Dr. Kuehn secured a St. Olaf Faculty Development Grant in 2014. The completion of multiple MCNER Research team local, national and international presentations followed. A publication related to faculty development implications derived from the MCNER full-scale study is in process. Collaboration through simulation on a small scale with nursing and social work students/faculty plus a chaplain and social work faculty has occurred. Future plans include incorporating pre-med students and a physician through a simulation with a patient in alcohol withdrawal.

Dr. Kuehn and Susan Huehn received the 2015 St. Olaf Academic Innovation Grant and a 2015 Sigma Theta Tau-Chi Chapter Research Scholarship to disseminate the findings. Dr. Kuehn participated in a recent National League of Nursing Scholarly Writing Retreat.

Nancy B. Leahy, RN, MSN, CHSE is an associate professor of nursing and simulation coordinator at John Tyler Community College in Richmond, Va. Ms. Leahy has worked as a nursing educator for more than 15 years and is currently enrolled in a doctoral program with a focus on nursing education. She participated in the first NLN Simulation Leadership cohort and has served on the Virginia State Simulation Alliance Board of Directors for 10 years. She has actively worked to support curriculum integration of simulation both locally and across the state of Virginia. Additionally, Ms. Leahy was appointed to the Virginia Community College System Curriculum Writing Team and has been working with other community college nurse educators to develop and implement a common curriculum for all state associate degree programs.

Nancy A. Maas, MSN, FNP-BC, CNE is an associate professor in the School of Nursing at Northern Michigan University, Marquette, Michigan. Ms. Maas has 23 years of experience as an RN in medical surgical nursing and has been a faculty member in both the LPN and BSN Programs at NMU for 12 years. She has served as the Simulation Education Coordinator for the School of Nursing since 2012, and has been instrumental in the expansion of the NMU simulation program and lab. Ms. Maas participated in the National League for Nursing Simulation Leadership Program in 2010 and has been involved in the development of simulation for health care education at the local and national levels.

Jeannette Manchester, DNP, RN is an assistant professor and the director for the Center for Professional Development at the Rutgers School of Nursing. Dr. Manchester was most recently the director of the Department of Education and Professional Development at University Hospital, in Newark, NJ, where she was responsible for operational leadership of the Department of Education at the hospital, overseeing the facilitation, organization, implementation, and evaluation of all staff education programs.

Prior to University Hospital, Dr. Manchester worked at the National League for Nursing, where she was the manager of professional development. While at the NLN, she directed all professional development activities, producing continuing education programs for faculty from conception to execution for all 34,000 members of the league across the country.

Dr. Manchester has also held positions as a nurse educator, critical-care transport nurse, and staff nurse for various health systems. She completed her DNP at UMDNJ, School of Nursing, and holds a master's in nursing education from Ramapo College, a BSN from Seton Hall University, and a BA in psychology from Rutgers University. She is currently pursuing her MBA at Rutgers School of Business.

Barbara McLaughlin, PhD, RN, CNE, ANEF is currently professor and head of the Department of Nursing at the Community College of Philadelphia. Dr. McLaughlin has been an associate degree nurse educator for over 30 years. She is a Certified Nurse Educator and a Fellow in the Academy of Nurse Educators. Since joining the full time faculty at Community College of Philadelphia, Dr. McLaughlin has participated in several grants, including the W. K. Kellogg Foundation funded Community College-Nursing Home Partnership to integrate gerontology into curricula and a Helene Fuld Health Trust grant related to refocusing associate degree nursing education into community based settings. Most recently she has participated in grants from The John A. Hartford Foundation and the Hearst Foundations, disseminating teaching strategies and evolving knowledge related to the care of older adults through activities related to Advancing Care Excellence for Seniors (ACE.S).

Heidi M. Meyer, MSN, RN, PHN is an associate professor of nursing at Gustavus Adolphus College. Her primary teaching responsibilities include health assessment, pharmacology, transitions to professional practice (senior capstone course), and integrating simulation throughout the curriculum. She also teaches a first term seminar on wellbeing. She serves as a faculty sponsor for nursing students completing independent research and has also been a faculty mentor for multiple nursing education graduate students. Her research interests include the scholarship of teaching and learning, specifically simulation in nursing education, emotional intelligence, and wellbeing.

MaryAnn McKenna Moon, MSN, APRN, ACNS-BC is the director of advanced practice nursing at Froedtert Memorial Lutheran Hospital in Milwaukee, WI. Ms. Moon is also an adjunct nursing professor at Minnesota State University in Mankato, Minnesota. She teaches health assessment and motivational interviewing to pre-licensure nursing students. Ms. Moon is focused on utilizing technology and simulation to enhance knowledge, clinical skills, and decision-making in both academic and health care settings. Her scientific interests include family engagement during chronic illness, proactive family care conferences in the ICU setting, care coordination, and transitions of care.

Diana Odland Neal, PhD, RN is an associate professor of nursing and chair of the Department of Nursing at St. Olaf College. Her educational background includes a BSN from St. Olaf College in Northfield, MN, a MS in Maternal-Child Health Nursing and Education from the University of Arizona in Tucson, AZ, and a PhD in Nursing from the University of Minnesota with a minor in Complementary Therapies and Healing Practices. Her clinical background is in neonatal intensive care unit (NICU) nursing, during which she worked as a staff nurse, transport nurse, and neonatal nurse educator. Dr. Neal also worked as the assistant nursing education coordinator at Children's Hospital in Minneapolis before beginning her teaching career in associate degree nursing at the College of St. Catherine (now St. Catherine's University) and in bachelor degree nursing at St. Olaf College for the past 20 years. She has publications focused on developmental care for preterm infants in the NICU and educational strategies related to teaching undergraduate nursing students. Dr. Neal is a member of the Minnesota Consortium for Nursing Education Research whose team received the 2012 Debra L. Spunt mini-grant for simulation research. Dr. Neal also received a Sigma Theta Tau Chi-At-Large Chapter Scholarship Award in 2013 and a Faculty Development Grant for simulation research from St. Olaf College in 2013.

Mary B. Reynolds, MSN/ED, RN is the director of quality assurance and compliance at Allay Home and Hospice, Inc. in Brookfield, WI. Her work has spanned oncology/hematology in all settings, home care, and hospice home care, and in the past 20 years she has been an adjunct associate professor and director of home and hospice care programs. She is a member of ANA, WNA, NLN and STTI.

Mary Anne Rizzolo, EdD, RN, FAAN, ANEF has focused her career on exploring new technologies, determining how they can inform and educate nurses, operationalizing their cost-effective delivery, and disseminating their value for education and practice. She pioneered the development of screen-based simulations that won national and international awards, and created one of the first websites in the world offering continuing education, journal articles, and networking opportunities for nurses. She has delivered over 250 national and international presentations, has served on many national committees and advisory boards, and is currently serving on the Society for Simulation in Healthcare's Board of Directors. During her tenure as a staff member at the National League for Nursing, Dr. Rizzolo managed all of the simulation projects. She now maintains an active consulting practice that includes managing several simulation projects for the National League for Nursing and others.

Colleen Royle, EdD, MSN, RN serves as the learning resource laboratory and simulation coordinator within the School of Nursing at Minnesota State University in Mankato, MN. Dr. Royle has presented her expertise in simulation and family nursing both nationally and internationally. In 2013, Dr. Royle and her colleagues were awarded the Hearst Foundations' Excellence in Geriatric Education Award for their work with the National League for Nursing (NLN) ACE.S Unfolding Cases. Dr. Royle is a member of the 2016 NLN Leadership Development Program for Simulation Educators cohort. Research interests include measuring the student preference of oral versus video-assisted debriefing, incorporating the process of family nursing into each simulation, and evaluating the teaching-learning experience for students and faculty.

Melanie Smerillo, MSN, RN, PHN is Co-Founder of Visual Medical, Inc. and a Registered Nurse at Children's Hospital of Minnesota. She received her MSN, with a concentration in Nursing Education, from St. Catherine University, where she worked as an assistant professor of nursing. Her areas of expertise and research include curriculum development, simulation, and clinical reasoning/critical thinking. In 2012, she co-founded Visual Medical, Inc., a medical device company in Minnesota whose mission is to develop world-class products using medically sound approaches while focusing on patient education, accessibility, and empowerment. She currently works as a hematology/oncology registered nurse at Children's Hospital of Minnesota.

Laureen Tavolaro-Ryley, MSN, RN, CNS is the independence foundation chair in nursing at Community College of Philadelphia, where she is a full-time faculty member and leads service learning collaboration between nursing students and the local community. She received her BSN from York College of Pennsylvania and an MSN in mental health nursing from the University of Pennsylvania School of Nursing, and a post master's certificate from the Psychiatric Mental Health Nurse Practitioner program at Drexel University. Ms. Tavolaro-Ryley has been involved with the ACE.S project since its inception as an expert in the field of geriatric mental health. She has been a featured speaker at the ACE.S conferences and webinars, has authored many of the ACE.S related teaching strategies, and is featured on the AJN's "How to Try This" series and the ACESXPRESS resource video. Ms. Tavolaro-Ryley has a private practice managing the mental health needs of geriatric clients, and serves as a legal consultant in cases involving geriatric clients.

Jone Tiffany, DNP, RN, RNC is a professor of nursing at Bethel University in St. Paul, MN. In her academic role, she is involved in the use of simulation in both the lab and virtual setting, and teaches nursing informatics. She also sits on the Board of Directors for the HealthEast Care system located in St. Paul, MN. She has presented nationally and internationally on the use of simulation to improve outcomes, and on the use of the virtual world Second Life® for nursing and medical education. Dr. Tiffany is the owner of two islands in the virtual world of Second Life®, where she is working on developing educational activities for healthcare students and professionals. Her Doctor of Nursing Practice system change project was titled: Second Life®: An Innovative Strategy for Teaching Inclusivity to Healthcare Professionals. Dr. Tiffany is a member of the Ramsey County Medical Reserve Corps, assisting with emergency preparedness training and giving immunizations in the community. She is also a Certified Gallup Strengthsfinder coach.

Stacey Van Gelderen, DNP, RN has been in clinical practice since 1999 and has been educating baccalaureate nursing students since 2005. She is a co-principal of multiple funded grants focusing on community and public health initiatives, as well as grants for developing wearable technology. She serves on the community leadership team for Martin, Faribault, & Watonwan counties in conjunction with the Minnesota State Health Improvement Program and is co-chair for the Madelia Community Based Collaborative. Her clinical expertise and interests include simulation in nursing education, maternal-child, family, community, and societal health. Dr. Van Gelderen developed the Van Gelderen Family Care Rubric to aid in improving nursing student communication and assessment skills of families through the use of simulation, and has been actively developing a family-focused electronic health record called Simulation, Analytics, and Family-focused Electronic Health Record (SAFEHR) designed to capture family health concerns, relationships, and resources to improve family health outcomes through wearable eyeglass technology for hands-free documentation and communication with families.

Lorrie Wong, PhD, RN, CHSE-A is the director of the University of Hawaii Translational Health Science Simulation Center and an associate professor at the University of Hawaii at Manoa School of Nursing and Dental Hygiene (UHSONDH), where she has taught since 1989. She received her PhD from the UHSONDH, her master's degree in nursing from Columbia University, and a bachelor's degree in nursing and post-master's certificate in adult advanced practice nursing from the UHSONDH. She is an adult advanced practice nurse with experience in critical care, intensive care, and trauma. In 2006, Dr. Wong was appointed as the Director for Simulation Learning, responsible for development of the University of Hawaii School of Nursing's simulation program and overseeing creation of the new state-of-the art translational health science simulation center. In 2010, she was selected to participate in the National League for Nursing Simulation Educator Program. Dr. Wong's research interests include integration of new technologies and teaching methodologies into health care education with a focus on interprofessional education, quality and patient safety, and clinical outcomes. In 2014, Dr. Wong was appointed to the College of Health Sciences and Social Welfare Interprofessional Education Workgroup.

Jean Ellen Zavertnik, DNP, RN, ACNS-BC, CNE is the simulation director at Clemson University School of Nursing. She has been in a faculty position for the last 10 years, with previous nursing experience in critical care. Dr. Zavertnik was among the first to participate in the National League for Nursing Leadership Development Program for Simulation Educators. She has published and presented on the use of simulation in nursing education.

Foreword

The late Dr. Andrea Mengel, to whom this book is dedicated, was a trailblazer in geriatric nursing and a devoted co-creator of the ACE.S project. In her decades-long career at the Community College of Philadelphia, Dr. Mengel reflected the best in nursing and nurse education. Her commitment to compassionate, informed nursing drove her and her colleagues to create a program that would fill the void in gerontological nursing content in curricula, expand faculty expertise in teaching gerontological nursing, and heighten students' experiences related to the care of older adults. The outcome was ACE.S.

ACE.S was created based on findings from a survey of nurse educators that indicated that new content needed to be accessible and seamlessly implemented within existing nursing curricula. Within this context, the ACE.S team cleverly developed a framework encompassing three essential knowledge domains and essential nursing actions. The three essential knowledge domains are individualized aging, complexity of care, and vulnerability during transitions. Beyond theory, students learn practice through unfolding cases and the essential nursing actions of assessment, coordinating care, using evolving knowledge, and making situational decisions.

By bringing the complexities of caring for aging patients to life through simulation scenarios within unfolding cases, the ACE.S program builds nursing judgment and prepares students for "the real world." We hope that the endearing unfolding cases of Millie Larsen, Red Yoder, and others, and the teaching moments surrounding them, help nurse educators across the nation share the challenges and joys of caring for aging patients.

To the nurse educators who have the opportunity in these pages to learn about ACE.S, teach the underlying academic theory, and expose students to the unfolding cases and simulations, the Hearst Foundations are grateful to you for your commitment to nursing education and to preparing the next generation of this noble workforce to care for older adults. Given the rapid growth of the senior population in the United States, it is imperative that our nurses, serving on the front lines of health care, have the most robust training possible.

ACE.S could not be what it has become today without Dr. Mengel and her colleagues' tireless efforts. We are delighted to see this major undertaking come to fruition, codifying the ACE.S work and perpetuating the field of geriatric nursing education that was so dear to Dr. Mengel.

George B. Irish
Eastern Director, Hearst Foundations
New York, New York

Preface

In early spring 2009, 10 nurse educators gathered at the Independence Foundation in Philadelphia to develop minimum standards for the integration of gerontological nursing content in nursing education. Dr. Andrea Mengel and I worked with them over the subsequent months to develop a framework for gerontological content alignment. A few months later, in Phoenix, AZ, Drs. Mary Anne Rizzolo and Pamela Jeffries met with a group of nurse educators who are experts in simulation to develop scenarios and unfolding cases to apply the framework. I have often reflected that both groups had no way of knowing the impact and reach of their work over the next five to six years.

This initial phase of development was funded by the John A. Hartford Foundation as a collaborative effort between the National League for Nursing (NLN) and Community College of Philadelphia (CCP). Independence Foundation, a private foundation in Philadelphia and CCP's funding partner, provided support for program evaluation, and Laerdal Medical Corporation provided support to develop simulations and unfolding case studies related to the care of older adults. Over the years, additional funders supported our efforts: the Hearst Foundations, the MetLife Foundation, and Independence Blue Cross Foundation of Southeast Pennsylvania.

Initially, we met in two groups whose members had in common a commitment to improving care for older adults and their caregivers, and teaching excellence. As I look back on those early days, I realize how quickly our two groups merged into one collaborative team. In selecting expert teachers for the team, we chose well. Our intention was that the outcomes of the project, known as ACE.S—Advancing Care Excellence for Seniors—would be evidence-based, teacher-ready tools that would fully engage students and faculty in the work of improving care for older adults. (The names of the faculty and staff that comprise the ACE.S team are listed in the Acknowledgments section later in the frontmatter.)

From these chaotic beginnings emerged the ACE.S framework and unfolding cases and teaching strategies, a model that has since been replicated with other populations. The NLN now offers ACE.Z, Advancing Care Excellence for Alzheimer's patients and their caregivers, as well as ACE.V, Advancing Care Excellence for Veterans, and we have plans to continue the series.

One cannot fully know how grants will evolve. From the beginning, we worked as a group of strangers from a broad set of objectives and embraced the ambiguity that goes with starting a new project without clear plans and directives. For all of us, it was a very special time. As the years unfolded and the project grew in dimension and impact, and the Hearst Foundations joined us to fund the wide dissemination of ACE.S, we traveled the country, creating stories that will live with us for a lifetime, and developed a bond that has been professionally meaningful for us all.

This book provides a roadmap for the development and implementation of ACE.S. The first section offers the foundational evidence for the ACE.S framework and evaluation of the total project; the second section presents exemplars of how faculty, many of them NLN Hearst Foundations Award winners, applied the ACE.S framework to their unique curricula. The book is a guide for faculty to study the underpinnings of the ACE.S framework as a foundation for use of the ACE.S resources provided for free on the NLN website (NLN.org/ACES). (Please note that many of the chapters in this publication were originally published by the NLN in the NLN journal *Nursing Education Perspectives.* Some have been revised and updated.)

For those of us committed to the care of vulnerable populations through excellence in nursing education, the journey continues. I am indebted to the ACE.S team for their unwavering commitment to this project and to the nurse educators who have shared their wisdom and experience in this book. I am also grateful to the educators from around the nation and the world who attended our workshops and webinars. The numbers far exceeded our initial projections and continue to grow, with traffic to the ACE.S section of the NLN website in the tens of thousands. Most important, I am gratified that nurse educators are embracing the comprehensive educational approach of the NLN ACE.S initiative and are teaching nursing students every day to provide safe, individualized, and high-quality care to older adults and their caregivers. Their work makes the journey extraordinary.

M. Elaine Tagliareni, EdD, RN, CNE, FAAN
*Chief Program Officer and Director of the
NLN Center for Excellence in the Care
of Vulnerable Populations*
National League for Nursing
Washington, DC

Acknowledgments: ACE.S Project Faculty and Staff (2009–2016)

The NLN is most grateful to the faculty and staff who co-created, implemented, evaluated, and disseminated ACE.S throughout this project. Their dedication to the project and commitment to excellence in the care for older adults is extraordinary.

Kellie Bassell, EdS, MSN, Chamberlain College of Nursing, IL

Teri Boese, MSN, RN, University of Texas at Arlington, TX

Tiffany Carson, NLN, NY (2013)

Mary Cato, EdD, RN, Oregon Health & Sciences University, OR

Jeanne Cleary, MA, RN, Ridgewater College, MN

Daniel D. Cline, PhD, RN, ANP-BC, Samuel Merritt University, CA

Martha A. Conrad, MSN, RN, University of Akron, OH

Tamika Curry, MSN, RN, Community College of Philadelphia, PA

Susan Gross Forneris, PhD, RN, CNE, CHSE-A, NLN, Washington, DC

Andrew Frados, MSN, RN, Miami Dade College, FL

Mary Gelbach, MSN, RN, Delaware County Community College, PA

Pamela Ironside, PhD, RN, FAAN, ANEF, Indiana University, IN

Pamela R. Jeffries, PhD, RN, FAAN, ANEF, George Washington University, Washington, DC

Eunice King, PhD, RN, Independence Foundation (Retired), Philadelphia, PA

Anita Kolvasky, MNEd, RN, Valencia Community College, FL

Barbara McLaughlin, PhD, RN, CNE, ANEF, Community College of Philadelphia, PA

Aida Mejia, NLN, NY (2012-2013)

Andrea Mengel, PhD, RN, Community College of Philadelphia, PA

Tatiana Nin, NLN, Washington, DC

Tricia O'Hara, PhD, RN, Gwynedd-Mercy College, PA

Cynthia Reese, PhD, RN, CNE, University of Illinois at Chicago, IL

Mary Anne Rizzolo, EdD, RN, FAAN, Consultant, NLN

Sheron Rowe, MSN, RN, LHRM, Seminole State College, FL

Leslie Sammarco, MSN, RN, Seminole State College, FL

Elaine Tagliareni, EdD, RN, CNE, FAAN, NLN, Washington, DC

Laureen Tavolaro-Ryley, MSN, RN, Community College of Philadelphia, PA

Naomi Wetmore, Community College of Philadelphia, PA

Contents

About the Editor   iv

About the Contributors   v

Foreword   xiii

Preface   xiv

Acknowledgments: ACE.S Project Faculty and Staff (2009–2016)   xvi

**SECTION 1   THE ACE.S FRAMEWORK: THEORETICAL
FOUNDATIONS   1**

CHAPTER 1   **Quality Care for Older Adults: The NLN Advancing Care
Excellence for Seniors (ACE.S) Project   3**
*M. Elaine Tagliareni, EdD, RN, CNE, FAAN, Daniel D. Cline, PhD, RN,
Andrea Mengel, PhD, RN, Barbara McLaughlin, PhD, RN, CNE, ANEF, and
Eunice S. King, PhD, RN*

CHAPTER 2   **A Concept Analysis of Individualized Aging   15**
Daniel D. Cline, PhD, RN

CHAPTER 3   **Complexity of Care: A Concept Analysis of Older Adult
Health Care Experiences   31**
Daniel D. Cline, PhD, RN

CHAPTER 4   **A Concept Analysis of Vulnerability During
Transitions   43**
Daniel D. Cline, PhD, RN

CHAPTER 5   **Gerontological Nursing Content in General Medical/
Surgical Textbooks: Where Is It?   55**
*Daniel D. Cline, PhD, RN, Jeannette Manchester, DNP, RN, and
M. Elaine Tagliareni, EdD, RN, CNE, FAAN*

CHAPTER 6   **Integrating QSEN and ACE.S: An NLN Simulation
Leader Project   67**
*Susan G. Forneris, PhD, RN, CNE, CHSE-A, JoAnn G. Crownover, DNP, RN,
CNE, Laurie Dorsey, MSN, RN, Nancy B. Leahy, RN, MSN, CHSE,
Nancy A. Maas, MSN, FNP-BC, CNE, Lorrie Wong, PhD, RN, CHSE-A,
Anne Zabriskie, MS, RN, CNE, and Jean Ellen Zavertnik, DNP, RN,
ACNS-BC, CNE*

CHAPTER 7   **ACE.S Program Evaluation: Faculty Use of the ACE.S Concepts and Resources   73**
Eunice S. King, PhD, RN

SECTION 2   APPLICATION OF ACE.S: TEACHING AND RESEARCH   85

CHAPTER 8   **ACE.S Teaching Resources for Classroom, Simulation and Clinical Practice   87**
M. Elaine Tagliareni, EdD, RN, CNE, FAAN, Mary Anne Rizzolo, EdD, RN, FAAN, ANEF, Laureen Tavolaro-Ryley, MSN, RN, CNS, and Tamika Curry, MSN, RN

CHAPTER 9   **Enhancing Clinical Reasoning Through Simulation Debriefing: A Multisite Study   95**
Susan G. Forneris, PhD, RN, CNE, CHSE-A, Diana Odland Neal, PhD, RN, Jone Tiffany, DNP, RN, RNC, Mary Beth Kuehn, EdD, RN, PHN, Heidi M. Meyer, MSN, RN, PHN, Linda M. Blazovich, DNP, RN, CNE, Ann E. Holland, PhD, RN, and Melanie Smerillo, MSN, RN, PHN

CHAPTER 10   **Clinical Application of ACE.S and the ACE.S Design Tree   107**
Michele Cislo, MA, RN

CHAPTER 11   **ACE.S Unfolding Case Simulations Redesigned to Address Family Nursing Care Competencies for Older Adults   113**
Norma Krumwiede, EdD, MEd, MN, RN, Colleen Royle, EdD, MSN, RN, Kelly Krumwiede, PhD, RN, PHN, Stacey Van Gelderen, DNP, RN, MaryAnn McKenna Moon, MSN, APRN, ACNS-BC, and Walter Groteluschen, MS

CHAPTER 12   **Thinking Like a Nurse: Optimizing Clinical Judgment and Reasoning Through the ACE.S Unfolding Cases   123**
Colleen Royle, EdD, MSN, RN, MaryAnn McKenna Moon, MSN, APRN, ACNS-BC, Norma Krumwiede, EdD, MEd, MN, RN, Stacey Van Gelderen, DNP, RN, Kelly Krumwiede, PhD, RN, PHN, and Walter Groteluschen, MS

CHAPTER 13   **A One-Day Geriatric Seminar Using ACE.S Resources   129**
Vivienne Friday, EdD, RN

CHAPTER 14   **Helping Students Process a Simulated Death Experience: Integration of an NLN ACE.S Evolving Case Study and the ELNEC Curriculum   133**
Judith A. Kopka, MSN, RN, CNE, Ann P. Aschenbrenner, PhD, RN, CNE, and Mary B. Reynolds, MSN/ED, RN

The ACE.S Framework: Theoretical Foundations

This section offers the foundational evidence for the ACE.S framework, including concept analyses of the ACE.S Essential Knowledge Domains, a discussion of the alignment of ACE.S to QSEN concepts, and a review of nursing education textbooks in relation to gerontology. The final chapter provides a comprehensive evaluation of the ACE.S Dissemination Project, funded by the Hearst Foundations; the impact of the ACE.S project nationally is discussed.

1

Quality Care for Older Adults: The NLN Advancing Care Excellence for Seniors (ACE.S) Project

M. Elaine Tagliareni, EdD, RN, CNE, FAAN

Daniel D. Cline, PhD, RN

Andrea Mengel, PhD, RN

Barbara McLaughlin, PhD, RN, CNE, ANEF

Eunice S. King, PhD, RN

ACE.S, the National League for Nursing's Advancing Care Excellence for Seniors project, is the first national effort to prepare students in all pre-licensure nursing programs to deliver high-quality care to older adults in a variety of settings. The project began as a partnership between the National League for Nursing (NLN) and Community College of Philadelphia. It was funded by the John A. Hartford Foundation, with additional support from Laerdal Medical, the Independence Foundation, and the Hearst Foundations. This chapter provides an overview of the ACE.S project and its guiding framework, which is intended for use by nurse educators in a variety of learning environments. The framework is designed to guide student experiences related to care of older adults and ultimately to promote quality care.

ACE.S was developed based on the premise that graduates of nursing programs must be competent in caring for multi-racial, multi-ethnic older adults and their families across multiple health settings (Institute of Medicine [IOM], 2011). A key component of ACE.S is that nursing students understand how older adults and their families interact with multiple health professionals along a continuum of care and how they make decisions about care before, during, and following life transitions. Coordinating care during significant life transitions is fundamental to ensuring competent, individualized, and humanistic care for older adults and their caregivers. Pre-licensure nursing education is central to ensuring that nurses understand and embrace these concepts.

BACKGROUND

For 20 years, national funders have advocated the integration of core content about nursing care of older adults into nursing school curricula. For example, the Robert

Wood Johnson Foundation (RWJF) funded the Teaching Nursing Home Project (1982–1987) to improve the quality of nursing home care and the clinical education of nurses by linking nursing schools with nursing homes (RWJF, 2011). The W.K. Kellogg Foundation funded the Community College Nursing Home Partnership grant (1986–1993) to enhance gerontological nursing education in associate degree programs (Waters, 1991).

Since 1996, the John A. Hartford Foundation, a leading philanthropic organization in the care of older adults, has funded programs related to advancing gerontological nursing at all levels of pre-licensure nursing education, as well as at the master's and doctoral levels, through initiatives administered by the American Academy of Nursing (AAN), the American Association of Colleges of Nursing (AACN), and the NLN. Funded programs have raised the visibility of gerontological nursing, improved gerontological nursing education, helped address the critical shortage of nursing leaders well versed in gerontological nursing research and education, and created several centers of gerontological nursing excellence (www.jhartfound.org).

Hartford Foundation projects have been funded to foster increased doctoral preparation of gerontological nurse researchers (Franklin et al., 2011), the development of multiple gerontological nursing resources through the Hartford Institute for Geriatric Nursing at New York University (http://hartfordign.org), and faculty development and leadership initiatives (Bednash, Mezey, & Tagliareni, 2011). Recently, the foundation expanded its focus to all pre-licensure nursing programs through the NLN ACE.S project. Through these efforts, the foundation has helped begin the transformation of gerontological nursing from an unnoticed specialty practice toward a practice that must be a core component of all nursing programs, both pre-licensure and post-baccalaureate.

Despite these concerted efforts by the Hartford Foundation and other philanthropic organizations to bring care of older adults to the forefront of nursing education, major gaps in pre-licensure nursing programs continue to exist. Specifically, programs lack gerontological nursing content in curricula, faculty expertise in knowledge related to care of older adults, and student experiences related to care of older adults. The ACE.S project aims to address these gaps. The project provides a foundation for nurse educators and students to advance care excellence for seniors in a variety of home, institutional, and community-based settings.

ACE.S is based on the NLN core values of caring, integrity, diversity, and excellence, and on the NLN Educational Competencies Model (2010b), which calls for graduates of nursing programs to be prepared to: a) promote and enhance human flourishing for patients, families, communities, and themselves; b) show sound nursing judgment; c) continually develop professional identity; and d) maintain a spirit of inquiry as they move into the world of nursing practice and beyond.

The NLN, through its *Reflection and Dialogue* series (NLN, 2010a), asked the nation's nurse educators to consider three essential questions to reframe thinking about care of older adults:

> ▸ As the number of older adults with acute and chronic conditions continues to increase, the goal of promoting health, function, quality of life, and end-of-life care provides complex challenges. Is this not a mandate to refocus and emphasize evidence-based care for older adults in nursing education curricula?

▸ What educational experiences are essential for preparing students to provide holistic, culturally competent, individualized care to older adults?

▸ How can faculty more effectively teach students to manage the complexity of care for older adults?

As the number of older patients with complex health needs increasingly outpaces the number of health care providers with the knowledge and skills to adequately care for them (IOM, 2008), the need to increase both the size and the capabilities of the existing nurse workforce to care effectively and efficiently for older adults is critical. This urgent national need drove the timely and innovative enrichments in nursing education promoted through the ACE.S project. The *NLN Vision Series,* "Caring for the Older Adult" (NLN, 2011), called on nurse educators nationally to better prepare students to advance the health of the nation's multi-ethnic, multi-racial older adult population. These calls for reform were designed to increase the nation's capacity to provide high-quality, affordable care to the rapidly growing older adult population. Additionally, the landmark Robert Wood Johnson Foundation funded Institute of Medicine report, *The Future of Nursing: Leading Change, Advancing Health* (2011), called for increased integration of gerontology and community-based care in pre-licensure curricula. Currently, pre-licensure nursing curricula "are not providing enough nurses with the required competencies in such areas as geriatrics and culturally relevant care to meet the changing health needs of the U.S. population" (IOM, 2011, 4–23). The IOM report also notes that the intricacies of care coordination are not adequately addressed in most pre-licensure nursing curricula. Taken together, these voices sounded a compelling argument for the transformation of nursing education.

ACE.S PROJECT DEVELOPMENT

Previous studies of baccalaureate nursing programs demonstrated a need for increased gerontological nursing content in pre-licensure curricula, as well as an increase in faculty with gerontological expertise (Berman et al., 2005; Gilje, Lacey, & Moore, 2007). However, no similar studies of the status of gerontological nursing content in other pre-licensure programs, associate degree and diploma, had been conducted. Therefore, in 2007, the John A. Hartford Foundation and the Independence Foundation of Philadelphia funded a project to assess how students in associate degree (AD) nursing programs were prepared to care for older adults. The project, *Fostering Geriatrics in Associate Degree Nursing Education,* was undertaken from 2007 to 2009 at Community College of Philadelphia in collaboration with the American Association of Community Colleges. The project was a multimethod study that included focus groups, an environmental scan, a national survey of the 851 AD nursing programs, and site visits to selected, geographically diverse AD schools (Ironside, Tagliareni, McLaughlin, King, & Mengel, 2010).

Findings from this study suggested that innovative approaches to faculty development were needed to update faculty expertise in gerontological nursing and in teaching strategies to enhance the preparation of pre-licensure students for the care of older adults. Strategies to enhance gerontological nursing content and experiences in pre-licensure programs needed to be readily accessible and easily implemented, with minimal additions to required faculty time and without adding content to already over-burdened curricula.

To that end, the NLN, Community College of Philadelphia, the Independence Foundation, and Laerdal Medical collaborated in the next phase of this project to: a) develop a set of guidelines to articulate the knowledge, skills, and attitudes essential in the care of older adults and required of all pre-licensure students entering the workforce, and b) to disseminate teaching strategies, tools, and resources for faculty in all pre-licensure RN programs. Dissemination of these resources would enable faculty to simultaneously strengthen their expertise in gerontological nursing and learn new ways of effectively and efficiently integrating this knowledge into their courses. This collaboration resulted in the creation of teaching strategies, several unfolding cases related to care of older adults, and the NLN ACE.S framework.

THE ACE.S FRAMEWORK

The NLN ACE.S framework evolved over time based on a review of the current literature, contributions from a panel of experts in education and gerontological nursing, and analysis of evaluation data following faculty development conferences attended by faculty from all types of pre-licensure nursing programs (AD, BSN, diploma). The framework identifies essential knowledge domains and essential nursing actions for pre-licensure nursing students. Rather than adding content to existing nursing curricula, the framework provides a context for the learning environment. (See Figure 1.1.)

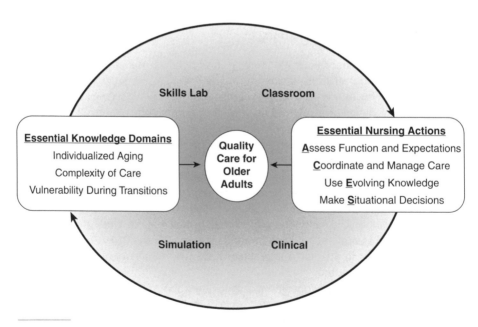

FIGURE 1.1 The National League for Nursing ACE.S Framework. (Copyright © 2012 by the National League for Nursing.)

Using the ACE.S framework as a guide, faculty plan and organize intentional student learning activities that build on the three components of the framework: the learning environment, essential knowledge domains and essential nursing actions. These three components lead to the framework's outcome: high-quality care for older adults in diverse health care and community settings. Incumbent in the framework is student acquisition of knowledge, skills, and attitudes related to quality care of older adults.

The Learning Environment

The context of the NLN ACE.S framework is the total learning environment experienced by students and faculty, including the classroom, skills laboratory, simulation lab, and direct patient care experiences. Learning activities focus on essential knowledge domains and essential nursing actions that are necessary for teaching care of older adults in ways that ensure students learn the complexities of this nursing specialty.

An important aspect of ACE.S is the use of simulation scenarios within unfolding cases to build bridges between and among the classroom, the simulation laboratory, and the clinical environment. The unfolding cases, introduced in compelling, first-person monologue stories, represent a range of challenges—medical, functional, psychosocial, and financial—typically faced by older adults. They are used by faculty as guides to develop encounters with older adults that incorporate all or some of the ACE.S essential nursing actions (King et al., 2011).

Use of the essential nursing actions in the classroom to guide learning objectives, and in the clinical setting to provide a framework for discussions during post-conference, helps students see connections between what is taught in lectures and the knowledge needed in clinical situations to deliver quality, safe nursing care. In summary, no learning experience is in isolation, and all learning experiences are viewed as interrelated.

ACE.S Essential Knowledge Domains

The three essential knowledge domains are individualized aging, complexity of care, and vulnerability during life transitions. Incorporation of these essential domains into pre-licensure nursing curricula will help students understand the lived experience of the older adult, as well as the challenges and rewards of caring for older adults.

Individualized Aging

The aging process is manifest and interpreted uniquely by each individual. Integral to the ACE.S concept of individualized aging is the understanding that there is no stereotypical way for older adults to age, both behaviorally and physiologically. Older adults live in a wide variety of settings and represent a broad spectrum of strengths, resources, needs, wishes, and expectations. The term, *individualized aging,* holds the promise of seeing each older adult as unique and requires nurses and all care providers to conduct a thorough and comprehensive assessment of each older adult for whom they provide care. This assessment allows the nurse to better understand how the older adult has internalized the lived experience of aging: What personal meaning does aging have?

What physiological changes have resulted from the aging process? What is the impact of those changes on activities of daily living (ADLs) and quality of life?

Conducting a comprehensive assessment of each older adult can have important clinical outcomes. For example, comprehensive geriatric assessments of hospitalized older adults conducted by multidisciplinary teams have demonstrated improved short-term mortality, better chances of living at home, and improved physical and cognitive functioning (Ellis & Langhorne, 2005). Important content areas that foster understanding of individualized aging may include: a) focused assessments (cognitive and functional abilities, geriatric syndromes, sexuality, nutrition, abuse and mistreatment, substance misuse), b) age-related changes, c) sensory changes, d) atypical presentations, e) oral health, and f) learning needs.

In Chapter 2 of this publication, Cline provides a concept analysis of individualized aging (Cline, 2014). The analysis discusses the heterogeneity of older adults, which is influenced by their past experiences and biological aging processes and contributes to variability in health outcomes. This fact is important for students to fully understand; often textbooks use the term "normal aging," which signifies to students that age-related changes are patterned, inevitable and most commonly lead to sequential decline. The concept of individualized aging creates a different perspective. It requires health care professionals to address the unique heterogeneous needs and preferences of older adult patients and refrain from applying clinical practice guidelines or protocols routinely, without accounting for difference and variability.

Complexity of Care

To manage the complex interplay of factors that influence quality care and quality of life, care of older adults requires specialized knowledge in both the art and science of gerontological nursing. Older adults represent a nurse's most complex clients, but this has not always been evident in how faculty teach care of older adults or in the experiences faculty create for students related to their care. Didactic and clinical experiences are needed to teach students to recognize, respect and respond to numerous interconnected factors that affect care and impact quality of life for older adults.

The management of multiple, co-existing acute and chronic conditions creates complex, clinically challenging situations. For example, hospitalized older adults are at increased risk for a variety of geriatric syndromes, which are multifactorial in nature and generally affect multiple organ systems (Inouye, Studenski, Tinetti, & Kuchel, 2007). Geriatric syndromes have serious consequences for older adults. Nurses educated to recognize the complex interplay of aging with acute and chronic conditions may be better prepared to prevent such complications.

Older adults' immediate and long-term life goals and physiological and mental health needs may converge in complex and unexpected ways as a result of changes in environments, levels of independence, and functional abilities. Nurse faculty must facilitate the ability of nurses to care for older adults and their caregivers in ways that recognize the complexity of care inherent in the aging process. Content areas for pre-licensure nursing programs that foster understanding of the complexity of care may include: a) geriatric syndromes (e.g., delirium, falls, incontinence, pressure ulcers, sleep disturbances),

b) oral hydration, c) fluid overload, d) infection, e) poly-pharmacy; f) depression, g) dementia, and h) multiple chronic diseases with acute exacerbations.

In Chapter 3 of this publication, Cline provides a concept analysis of complexity of care. The analysis calls out that complexity of care directly affects older adults by having positive or negative impacts on their quality of life and the quality of the care they receive (Cline, 2015). It is critically important for nurse educators to understand that simply telling students that care of older adults is complex does little to help them understand the concept. Using the ACE.S framework as a guide, nurse educators are able to assist students to understand the implications of complexity and the ways in which complexity can improve as well as diminish an older adult's life. Most importantly, nursing students need to recognize that complexity itself is neither bad nor good; rather, what is important is to *manage* complexity.

Vulnerability during Life Transitions

Aging is a dynamic process and an older adult is likely to make many transitions from one form, state, activity, or place to another. These transitions have the potential to create upheaval and disequilibrium for the older adult and the family. Coordinating care and advocating for the older adult during significant life transitions are fundamental to providing competent, individualized, humanistic care for the older adult, the family, and caregivers. Care must be more than a series of discrete services; rather, there must be continuity of care as the older adult moves among care settings. Evidence from the Transitional Care Model, developed by a multidisciplinary team at the University of Pennsylvania, has demonstrated the important role nurses have in mitigating vulner-abilities and improving outcomes for vulnerable older adults transitioning from acute care services to home (Naylor et al., 2004).

Integral to ensuring quality care is the nurse's understanding that older adults are vul-nerable during all transitions, whether the transition is from acute-care to rehabilitation settings, community to long-term care, or from complete independence with ADLs to dependence on others. Content areas for the pre-licensure nursing programs that foster understanding of the vulnerability during life transitions include: a) health care decision-making (culture, religion/spirituality, lived experiences, patient and family wishes and expectations, advanced directives), b) palliative care (hospice, end-of-life), c) iatrogen-esis, d) advocacy, e) environments of care (acute, community, long-term care, assisted living), f) interdisciplinary collaboration, and g) ageism. Pre-licensure nursing programs that integrate the ACE.S Essential Knowledge Domains into their curricula will provide students with crucial knowledge related to quality care of older adults.

In Chapter 4 of this publication, Cline provides a concept analysis of vulnerability during life transitions, defining vulnerability during transitions for older adults as the inadequate continuity of care and poor communication and coordination among health care providers and patients and their families (Cline, 2016). Coordinating care and advo-cating for the older adult during significant life transitions are fundamental to the ACE.S approach to delivery of competent, individualized, humanistic care for the older adult, the family, and caregivers. In fact, ACE.S's asks faculty and students to reframe their thinking about discharge, recognizing that older adults are never fully released or dis-charged from the health care delivery system. Using ACE.S as a framework suggests that health care providers no longer use the term *discharge planning* and consider *transition planning* as a more active and realistic alternative. In clinical teaching settings, for example, where older adults are discharged to home, nursing students would ensure that patients have a clear understanding of their medications and follow-up appointments with their primary care providers and that their caregivers have adequate support and guidance.

ACE.S Essential Nursing Actions

The essential nursing actions allow nursing students and practicing nurses to translate their knowledge of individualized aging, complexity of care, and vulnerabilities during life transitions into actions that promote high-quality care for older adults. Further, use of these essential nursing actions in clinical experiences, skills lab/simulation, and lecture develops knowledge, skills, and abilities related to the care of older adults while promoting positive perceptions of aging.

The ACE.S essential nursing actions build upon the existing Hartford-Foundation-funded resources and competencies to promote competent, individualized, and humanistic care for older adults. Central to this intent is a keen understanding that direct knowledge of older adults in planned, intentional encounters is necessary for nurses to promote human flourishing and sound nursing judgment. Use of the essential nursing actions helps faculty teach students how to provide quality care for older adults. It involves the development of nursing judgment and teaching students to notice what is happening by assessing the older adult's functional status; strengths, resources, needs, and cultural traditions; and the wishes and expectations of the older adult and caregiver. The teacher and student use evolving evidence-based geriatric knowledge, technology, and best practices to encourage a spirit of inquiry and provide competent care for the older adult. See Table 1.1.

Assess Function and Expectations

Teaching physical assessment is foundational in pre-licensure nursing programs. However, the inclusion of functional assessment skills, together with communication skills, to recognize, respond to, and respect an older adult's wishes and expectations has not always been included in comprehensive assessment courses. The assessment of an older adult's cognition and mood, as well as physical status and comfort, is essential to an understanding of individualized aging. In fact, the addition of functional assessment and focused communication to determine the older adult's, or caregiver's, wishes and expectations about treatment options and living arrangements has the potential to significantly improve quality of life.

Nursing actions call for a more comprehensive approach to assessment, one that utilizes standardized assessment tools, like the "How to Try This Series" (www.ConsultGeriRN.org), to create a baseline of functional and psychosocial abilities. Together with physical assessment findings, the inclusion of function and personal expectations and wishes helps gain a comprehensive view of the older adult's status. This interplay of assessment findings is essential to ensure the understanding of individualized aging.

TABLE 1.1

The National League for Nursing ACE.S Essential Nursing Actions

The Essential Nursing Actions enable nursing students and practicing nurses to translate their knowledge of individualized aging, complexity of care, and vulnerabilities during life transitions into actions that promote high quality care for older adults. Use in clinical experiences, skills lab/ simulation, and lecture develops students' knowledge, skills, and abilities related to the care of older adults, while promoting positive perceptions of aging.

Assess Function and Expectations	• Assess, respond to, and respect an older adult's functional status and strengths, wishes, and expectations. • Determine the older adult's function and expectations, along with cognition, mood, culture, physiologic status, and comfort to obtain a comprehensive assessment of health care needs. • Use standardized assessment tools to assess the older adult's individual aging pattern.
Coordinate and Manage Care	• Manage chronic conditions, including atypical presentations, in daily life and during life transitions to maximize function and maintain independence. • Assist older adults and families/caregivers to access knowledge and evaluate resources. • Advocate during acute exacerbations of chronic conditions to prevent complications.
Use Evolving Knowledge	• Understand geriatric syndromes and unique presentations of common diseases in older adults. • Access and use emerging information and research evidence about the special care needs of older adults and appropriate treatment options. • Interpret findings and evaluate clinical situations in order to provide high quality nursing care based on current knowledge and best practices.
Make Situational Decisions	• Analyze risks and benefits of care decisions in collaboration with the interdisciplinary team and the older adult, family, and caregivers. • Evaluate situations where standard treatment recommendations need to be modified to manage care in the context of the older adult's needs and life transitions. • Consider the older adult's wishes, expectations, resources, lived experiences, culture, and strengths when modifying care approaches.

Coordinate and Manage Care

Today, more than four out of five older adults experience one or more chronic conditions (AARP Public Policy Institute, 2009). People with chronic disease may have difficulty with basic ADLs, such as bathing, dressing, and eating; have significantly higher rates of hospitalization; and make more emergency room visits. Much of the demand for increased services in the hospital, outpatient, and emergency departments "will be driven by the growth in the absolute number of older Americans, which will result in a greater total volume of illness and disability and a greater collective need for services from the health care system" (IOM, 2008, p. 65).

When older adults enter the health care system for an acute exacerbation of a chronic condition, they require complicated and intense health care to not only restore health but to stabilize other chronic health problems. Management of chronic conditions includes an understanding of atypical presentations, as well as consideration of life transitions in order to maximize function and maintain the older adult's independence and quality of life.

Rarely does an older adult experience just one health care issue. For example, an older adult who is admitted to the hospital with a cardiac event may also have diabetes and arthritis, and may have experienced a stroke causing limited mobility and reduced bowel and bladder control. Nurses caring for this individual must address the acute issue of cardiac decompensation, while meeting needs related to the control of hyperglycemia and the pain of arthritis, as well as assisting the older adult to maintain functional ability related to mobility and continence.

During interviews conducted by project staff, students confirmed the need to address the complexity involved in care of older adults: "Our textbook is divided into sections and each one has a box with 'implications for the geriatric client.' So when you read about hip replacement, there is a box about caring for an elderly person with hip replacement. But we don't ever see a patient with a hip replacement. We see a patient with a hip replacement and hypertension and diabetes and . . ."

Managing chronic illnesses also involves assisting caregivers and families in accessing and evaluating resources. This aspect of care is often overlooked; in an AARP study, about two thirds of caregivers reported that the health of the person they assisted has worsened because he or she did not get the care needed (AARP, 2009). Essential nursing actions related to chronic care management is critical to fully be an advocate for older adults, to prevent complications, and to coordinate care across health care settings.

Use Evolving Knowledge

New knowledge related to care of older adults has emerged over the past several years. This evolving knowledge, particularly geriatric syndromes and atypical presentations, is vital information for faculty to acquire and pass on to students. Helping students to recognize, assess for, and prevent the untoward effects of geriatric syndromes will increase their understanding of the complexity of care inherent with older adults. The use of assessment tools that help nurses identify older adults at risk for geriatric syndromes will result in an increase in quality of life and assist older adults in transitioning from setting to setting.

An example would be discussing assessment and treatment of delirium, dementia, and depression in the older adult. An older adult with an existing dementia, for example, may also develop delirium. Students need to be able to assess the baseline dementia and recognize the onset of new behaviors. In addition, since delirium is usually a behavior associated with a physiological cause, such as urinary tract infection, it is important for the student to be able to assess for this and recognize the atypical presentation.

Make Situational Decisions

Taking into account the complexity of care involved with older adults, students need to be able to evaluate individual situations and analyze the risks and benefits of decisions.

The expectations and wishes of the older adult and the family need to be considered. Sometimes, the quality of life of the older adult is impacted negatively in the name of safety. Examples of situational decision-making occur frequently in health care. One client may choose to not have a treatment or procedure because the side effects will adversely affect quality of life, while another client, in a similar situation, will agree to the treatment or procedure. An elderly client may be safe riding a bicycle while another elderly client may not be safe.

Helping the older adult gather information and understand the risks and benefits associated with treatment options and life choices is a valuable nursing intervention. Nurses can help clients weigh the risks and benefits of impending decisions. Making informed choices, consistent with the client's preferences, culture, and values, is essential for quality nursing care.

WORKING TOWARD IMPROVED CARE OF OLDER ADULTS

An essential goal for the future must be to make the older adult the prototype client in nursing education. This approach would include conveying to students an understanding of how multiple chronic conditions create gaps in the quality and delivery of health care for older adults, and that promotion of improved functional status, quality of life, and maintenance of chronic conditions results in a more efficient and effective care system through better coordinated care and smooth transitions. To reach that goal, it is imperative that nurse educators create a nursing workforce with an appreciation and ability to apply the emerging body of knowledge associated with care of older adults in a wide variety of environments, including hospitals, rehabilitation centers, long-term care facilities, the older adult's home, and community care settings. ACE.S is designed to facilitate the realization of this goal.

Through the NLN website (www.NLN.org/ACES), curriculum tools such as simulations, unfolding cases, and teaching strategies continue to be widely circulated. The dissemination of ACE.S expanded, with funding from the Hearst Foundations, through one-day workshops focused on teaching faculty the essential knowledge domains and essential nursing actions, how to use unfolding cases and simulation, and how to champion effective organizational change to build a strong nursing workforce to deliver high-quality care to older adults. In Chapter 7 of this publication, King provides a comprehensive analysis of the ACE.S dissemination program, funded by the Hearst Foundation, describing how faculty used the ACE.S concepts and resources.

The NLN ACE.S project is designed to assist faculty to enhance their knowledge of the growing body of evidence about specialized care for older adults. ACE.S is based on a staunch belief that familiarity with the field of gerontology creates exciting learning opportunities for faculty, students, and their clinical partners. Central to this tenet is a keen understanding that direct knowledge of older adults in planned, intentional encounters with students is necessary in order for nurses to promote human flourishing with scientifically grounded nursing judgment and plan individualized, humanistic care for older adults and their caregivers.

References

AARP Public Policy Institute. (2009). *Chronic care: A call to action for health care reform.* Retrieved from http://assets.aarp.org/rgcenter/health/beyond_50_hcr.pdf

Bednash, G., Mezey, M., & Tagliareni, E. (2011). The Hartford Geriatric Nursing Initiative experience in geriatric nursing education: Looking back, looking forward. *Nursing Outlook, 59*(4), 228–241. doi: 10.1016/j.outlook.2011.05.012.

Berman, A., Mezey, M., Kobayashi, M., Fulmer, T., Stanley, J., & Thornlow, D. (2005). Gerontological nursing content in baccalaureate nursing programs: Comparison of findings from 1997 and 2003. *Journal of Professional Nursing, 21*(5), 268–275. doi:10.1016/j.profnurs.2005.07.005

Cline, D. D. (2014). A concept analysis of individualized aging. *Nursing Education Perspectives: 35* (3), 185–192.

Cline, D. D. (2015). Complexity of care: A concept analysis of older adult health care experiences. *Nursing Education Perspectives: 36*(2), 108–112.

Cline, D. D. (2016). A concept analysis of vulnerability during transitions. *Nursing Education Perspectives: 37*(2), 91–96.

Ellis, G., & Langhorne, P. (2005). Comprehensive geriatric assessment for older hospital patients. *British Medical Bulletin, 71*(1), 45–59. doi: 10.1093/bmb/ldh033

Franklin, P. D., Archbold, P. G., Fagin, C. M., Galik, E., Siegel, E., Sofaer, S., & Firminger, K. (2011). Building academic geriatric nursing capacity: Results after the first 10 years and implications for the future. *Nursing Outlook, 59*(4), 198–205. doi:10.1016/j.outlook. 2011.05.011

Gilje, F., Lacey, L., & Moore, C. (2007). Gerontology and geriatric issues and trends in U.S. nursing programs: A national survey. *Journal of Professional Nursing, 23*(1), 21–29. doi:10.1016/j.profnurs.2006.12.001

Inouye, S. K., Studenski, S., Tinetti, M. E., & Kuchel, G. A. (2007). Geriatric syndromes: Clinical, research, and policy implications of a core geriatric concept. *Journal of the American Geriatrics Society, 55*(5), 780–791. doi: 10.1111/j.1532–5415.2007.01156.x

Institute of Medicine. (2008). *Retooling for an aging America. Building the health care workforce.* Washington, DC: National Academies Press.

Institute of Medicine (2011). *The future of nursing: leading change, advancing health.* Washington, DC: National Academies Press.

Ironside, P. M., Tagliareni, M. E., McLaughlin, B., King, E., & Mengel, A. (2010). Fostering geriatrics in associate degree nursing education: an assessment of current curricula and clinical experiences. *Journal of Nursing Education, 49*(5), 246–252. doi:10.3928/01484834–20100217–01

King, E., Cline, D., Mengel, A., McLaughlin, B., Rizzolo, M. A., & Tagliareni, E. (2011). *Advancing Care Excellence for Seniors (ACES).* [Headlines from the NLN]. *Nursing Education Perspectives, 32*(4), 276–277.

The National League for Nursing. (2010a). Care of older Adults [Reflection and Dialogue]. Retrieved from www.nln.org/aboutnln/reflection_dialogue/refl_dial_5.htm

The National League for Nursing. (2010b). *Outcomes and competencies for graduates of practical/vocational, diploma, associate degree, baccalaureate, master's, practice doctorate, and research doctorate programs in nursing.* New York: Author.

The National League for Nursing. (2011). Caring for older adults [NLN Vision Series]. Retrieved from http://www.nln.org/aboutnln/livingdocuments/pdf/nlnvision_2.pdf

Naylor, M. D., Brooten, D. A., Campbell, R. L., Maislin, G., McCauley, K., & Schwartz, S. (2004). Transitional care of older adults hospitalized with heart failure: A randomized, controlled trial. *Journal of the American Geriatrics Society, 52*(5), 675–684. doi: 10.1111/j.1532–5415.2004.52202.x

Robert Wood Johnson Foundation. (2011). Nursing homes affiliated with nursing schools improve care [Teaching Nursing Home Project]. Retrieved from www.rwjf.org/files/research/26434.final.pdf

Waters, V. (Ed.). (1991). *Teaching gerontology.* New York: NLN Press.

2

A Concept Analysis of Individualized Aging

Daniel D. Cline, PhD, RN

ABSTRACT

AIM: This analysis sought to define the concept of individualized aging.

BACKGROUND: The increasing older adult population and the shortage of health professionals with adequate knowledge of their specialized needs will strain the health care system. The National League for Nursing's Advancing Care Excellence for Seniors (ACE.S) project has addressed this challenge. The ACE.S framework identifies three unique concepts integral to delivering high-quality care. Clarification of these concepts is needed for educational and research purposes.

METHOD: Rogers and Knafl's evolutionary method of concept analysis was used.

RESULTS: The analysis identified two antecedents (past experiences and biological aging processes), three attributes (heterogeneity, living with age-related changes and multiple chronic conditions, and risk for complications), and two consequences (complexity of care over time and variability in health outcomes).

CONCLUSION: Knowledge of the antecedents, attributes, and consequences of individualized aging will allow health care providers to improve the care of older adults.

The rapidly aging older adult population (those ages 65 years and older) combined with a lack of health care providers who possess the necessary knowledge, skills, and attitudes (Institute of Medicine [IOM], 2008) to provide high-quality care to this population is a concerning challenge that the profession of nursing must address (Berman et al., 2005; Gilje, Lacey, & Moore, 2007; Ironside, Tagliareni, McLaughlin, King, & Mengel, 2010). Nurses represent the largest segment of health care providers in the country and assume crucial roles in the care and management of both healthy and ill older adults. As the older-adult population grows, nurses will be expected to advance their roles and responsibilities in caring for these patients in a variety of settings, from home to hospital, as well as from assisted living to long-term care (IOM, 2011).

BACKGROUND

In the past several years, significant efforts have been made to improve the quality of gerontological nursing content in nursing education programs at both the pre-licensure level (American Association of Colleges of Nursing [AACN], 2010; the National League for Nursing [NLN], 2011) and at the graduate level (National Council of State Boards of Nursing, 2008). The John A. Hartford Foundation (JAHF) has been a generous supporter of efforts aimed at improving gerontological nursing education and research, and several of its funded initiatives (Building Academic Geriatric Nursing Capacity Program—now called the National Hartford Centers of Gerontological Nursing Excellence—and the Hartford Institute for Geriatric Nursing) have led to significant increases in faculty with expertise in gerontological nursing and programs of research aimed at improving the care of older adults (Franklin et al., 2011). The JAHF also partnered with the AACN to create the *Recommended Baccalaureate Competencies and Curricular Guidelines for the Nursing Care of Older Adults* (2010) as a supplement to *The Essentials of Baccalaureate Education for Professional Nursing Practice.*

An NLN vision statement, *Caring for Older Adults* (2011), describes the NLN's vision for transforming nursing education to enhance the knowledge, skills, and attitudes of graduate nurses caring for older adults. In 2007, the NLN, in collaboration with the Community College of Philadelphia and funded by the Independence Foundation, the JAHF, Laerdal Medical, and, since 2012, the Hearst Foundations, began developing the Advancing Care Excellence for Seniors (ACE.S) project and the ACE.S framework to improve the care of older adults (Tagliareni, Cline, Mengel, McLaughlin, & King, 2012).

The ACE.S framework, designed for use in pre-licensure nursing education programs, is also applicable to graduate nursing programs and other health care disciplines. The framework has three primary components that interact synergistically to improve the quality of care for older adults: essential knowledge domains, essential nursing actions, and learning environment.

The NLN ACE.S framework's essential knowledge domains (individualized aging, complexity of care, and vulnerability during transitions) may be unfamiliar to nurse clinicians, educators, and researchers. Although these basic concepts are commonly found in the health sciences literature, their precise definitions and descriptions within the NLN ACE.S framework are unique. Explication of these concepts will advance the use of the ACE.S framework, improve gerontological nursing education, and facilitate the design of research aimed at improving the quality of care for older adults.

Individualized aging is a concept not currently used or defined in the literature. However, it is well established that high-quality care must be individualized so that each patient receives treatments appropriate to his or her needs and desires and that it be based on the best available evidence to ensure optimal outcomes. Individualized aging synthesizes concepts of individualization of care as well as biological and social theories related to the aging process. By using concept analysis, this article will define and clarify the NLN ACE.S framework essential knowledge domain concept of individualized aging.

METHOD

The evolutionary method of concept analysis (Rogers & Knafl, 2000) focuses on the concept's contextual and temporal nature, which is appropriate to this analysis given the rapid technological advances in health care and society that have prolonged and improved the quality of life for older adults beyond what was possible even two decades ago. The goal of concept analysis (Rogers & Knafl, 2000) is to identify a set of attributes that "constitute a real definition" (p. 91), making it possible to identify situations that can be appropriately characterized by the concept.

Sample

Two approaches were used to identify the relevant literature. The first approach was designed to identify current information on biological and psychosocial theories of aging. Four nursing textbooks, two published in 2010 and two in 2012, were examined to identify the most commonly described theories of aging. The second approach focused on identifying literature on the concept of individualized care from the fields of nursing, medicine, and social work. Because the ACE.S project began in 2007, the electronic databases of PubMed®, CINAHL®, and Web of Science™ were searched from the years 2007 through 2012. Inclusion criteria included publication in an English-language, peer-reviewed journal. Exclusion criteria included editorials, published abstracts, and commentaries. To search the literature systematically, the term "individualized care" was combined with "older adult(s)," "geriatric(s)," "elderly," and "aging."

A total of 334 articles were identified in the initial search. Review of the abstracts for duplicate articles and for inclusion and exclusion criteria reduced the final analytic sample to 146 articles. Twenty percent of the total population of articles, or at least 30 articles, whichever is greater, provides a sample of adequate size to conduct an analysis (Rogers and Knafl, 2000). Therefore, 30 of the 146 articles were selected for inclusion in this analysis.

Data Analysis

Individualized aging is a compound concept, meaning that each word in the concept has meaning. Analysis proceeded first by analyzing data on current theories of aging and was followed by reviewing the sample of scientific articles for data on individualized care. Many articles did not forthrightly define the concept of individualized care; rather, aspects of the concept were referred to in the articles' introductions as a finding or result, or in discussion sections. Rogers and Knafl (2000) indicate that the absence of a definition is common and recommend looking for statements on characteristics of the concept while keeping in mind how the concept is used in practice. They also recommend that researchers "look for all statements that provide a clue to how the author defines the concept" (p. 91). Data elements of current theories of aging and data elements from each article were extracted into a table for inductive analysis, a key component of the evolutionary method of concept analysis (Rogers & Knafl, 2000), to identify the attributes, antecedents, and consequences of the concept being analyzed.

FINDINGS

Analysis of the data revealed two antecedents, three defining attributes, and two consequences (see Figure 2.1). Specific textual data from the sample articles were used as examples of each of the attributes, antecedents, and consequences discussed.

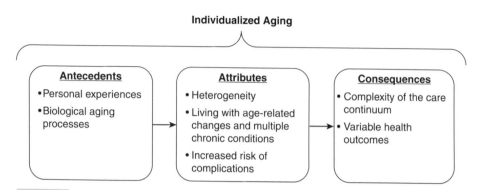

FIGURE 2.1 Antecedents, attributes, and consequences of individualized aging.

Antecedents

Antecedents are phenomena or events that occur prior to the concept (Rogers & Knafl, 2000), but are an integral part of it. The two antecedents identified as preceding the concept of individualized aging were past experiences and biological aging processes.

Past Experiences

Older adults' past experiences influence their beliefs, attitudes, expectations, and interactions with the health care system and health care professionals. Psychological and sociological theories of aging (e.g., activity, disengagement, gerotranscendence, age stratification) help explain the impact of past experiences on older adults and subsequently on the process of aging. The activity theory (Havighurst, 1961) suggests that older adults' continued engagement with society through activities they enjoyed in middle age promotes both psychosocial and physical well-being. Older adults viewed through this theoretical lens might be more likely to have increased functional ability and to want more aggressive treatment options for illness and injury even if the prognosis is potentially poor, as with some types of cancer.

Disengagement theory (Cumming & Henry, 1961) posits that as people age they gradually disengage from society to make room for younger people to take over the primary responsibilities of society, thereby maintaining societal equilibrium. Older adults viewed through this theoretical lens might be more likely to have less functional ability and to not choose aggressive treatment options. Gerotranscendence (Tornstam, 1994) theory also predicts a natural disengagement from society, but holds that this is positive, because older adults can then focus on metaphysical needs and introspection.

Another theory, age stratification (Riley, Johnson, & Foner, 1972), looks at older adults as cohorts of similar-age individuals creating varying strata within society. These strata or cohorts share common past experiences, such as living through World War II or the civil rights era, that shape their views and expectations as well as society's views and expectations of them. The current stratum of baby boomers in the United States may bring significant changes to how the country's health care system functions as a result of their past experiences. This generation of older adults is expected to have better health and therefore longer lives and to be better educated, more connected to society, and more personally involved in health care decisions than any previous cohort.

Biological Aging Processes

All living organisms experience cellular degradation and decline that lead to death (Eliopoulos, 2010; Maulk, 2010; Miller, 2012; Touhy & Jett, 2012). The rate and effects of decline are different for each individual. Several theories hypothesize the underlying mechanisms of cellular decline based on knowledge and examination of the organism's genetic makeup and cellular activities. For example, the neuroendocrine and immunological theories of aging posit that the diminished abilities of these body systems contribute to biological aging (Fabris, 1991). Loss of the neuroendocrine system's ability to release hormones secreted by various endocrine glands contributes to cells' inability to function normally, leading to cellular and organ decline—thereby influencing the aging process. It is also theorized that impaired immunological processes contribute to the aging process and lead to increased disease in older adults (Swain & Nikolich-Zugich, 2009).

The free radical theory of aging posits that highly unstable and reactive molecules, called *free radicals,* damage cells (Harman, 1956). Although the body has protective mechanisms against these molecules, their effectiveness declines over time and the cellular damage accumulates, contributing to the aging process. Biological decline appears to be part of the aging process; however, each individual's rate of decline, based on factors identified in current biological theories of aging, impacts the individual aging process. Biological decline is intricately linked to each individual's past experiences, creating a unique process. Past experiences also interact synergistically with individualized biological decline processes, leading to an individualized aging process.

Attributes

There are three attributes of individualized aging: heterogeneity, living with age-related changes and chronic conditions, and increased risk for complications.

Heterogeneity

The first attribute of individualized aging is the recognition that the older adult population in the United States is extremely heterogeneous—diverse—in many different ways. The reviewed articles (see Table 2.1) frequently discussed this heterogeneousness in physiological variables, cultural preferences, racial/ethnic disparities, and response to illness. For example, Studenski and colleagues (2011) found that gait speed and life expectancy vary widely among older adults. Gait speed can range from 0.04 m/s to 1.4 m/s and life expectancy for those 70 years old varies between 7 and 23 years for men and 10 and 33 years for women, and there is an association between gait speed and life expectancy. The heterogeneity seen in older adults' life expectancy creates a need to consider this reality when individualizing treatment plans (Studenski et al., 2011). This is also significant because quality of life is increased when treatment plans are individualized (Parsons, Rouse, Robinson, Sheridan, & Connolly, 2012).

TABLE 2.1

Literature on Attributes of Individualized Aging

Attribute	Author(s), Year
Heterogeneity	Ahalt et al., 2012 American Geriatrics Society, 2012b Bielaszka-DuVernay, 2011 Bowling & O'Hare, 2012 Bradway et al., 2011 Curtiss, 2010 Feldblum et al., 2011 Germino, 2011 Krall et al., 2012 Lewis et al., 2009 Ligthelm et al., 2012 Maynard et al., 2008 Nitz et al., 2011 Parsons et al., 2012 Studenski et al., 2011 Szanton et al., 2011 Tamura et al., 2012 Tjia et al., 2008
Living with Age-Related Changes and Multiple Chronic Conditions	Ahalt et al., 2012 Almeida et al., 2012 American Geriatrics Society, 2012a Balducci et al., 2010 Bielaszka-DuVernay, 2011 Bowling & O'Hare, 2012 Bradway et al., 2011 Curtiss, 2010 Krall et al., 2012 Lewis et al., 2009 Ligthelm et al., 2012 Lorenz et al., 2012 Mänty et al., 2009 Maynard et al., 2008 Planton & Edlund, 2009 Richards et al., 2011 Wang et al., 2012
Increased Risk of Complications	Almeida et al., 2012 American Geriatrics Society, 2012a Curtiss, 2010 Feldblum et al., 2011 Germino, 2011 Krall et al., 2012 Lakatos et al., 2009 Ligthelm et al., 2012 Maynard et al., 2008 McCurry et al., 2012 Nitz et al., 2011 Planton & Edlund, 2009

Heterogeneity is also seen in the desire of older adults of differing racial or ethnic groups to discuss health care prognoses with their providers and the view "that a doctor should not make assumptions based on ethnicity" (Ahalt et al., 2012, p. 572), emphasizing their desire to be viewed as individuals even within a specific cultural or ethnic group. Older adults' cultural and ethnic backgrounds can also affect how they age and interpret past experiences. Szanton and colleagues (2011) focused on improving older African-Americans' ability to age in place in recognition of their increased rates of disease and disability as well as their lower socioeconomic status (SES) compared to their white counterparts. Heterogeneity of SES is an important component of older adults' past experiences that impacts how they age.

The American Geriatrics Society (AGS) emphasizes that "older adults with multimorbidity are heterogeneous in terms of illness severity, functional status, prognosis, personal priorities, and risk of adverse events even when diagnosed with the same pattern of conditions" (2012b, p. 1957). The literature identifies the need for changes in care guidelines in at least two areas—diabetes (Germino, 2011; Ligthelm, Kaiser, Vora, & Yale, 2012) and renal disease (Bowling & O'Hare, 2012; Campbell & O'Hare, 2008; Tamura, Tan, & O'Hare, 2012)—due to the heterogeneous nature of older adults. Standardized treatments (for, e.g., diabetes and renal care) applied without consideration of the diverse and unique needs of older adults may not be appropriate and may contribute to poor outcomes and diminished quality of life.

Many older adults with adequate functional status and social support live long, productive lives. Age alone should not determine treatment plans; rather, each older adult's functional status, social situation, and health status should be considered because they all contribute to the likelihood of older adults living healthy, productive lives.

Living With Age-Related Changes and Chronic Conditions

A second attribute of individualized aging is the reality that older adults live with multiple age-related physiological changes and multiple chronic conditions. "One of the greatest challenges in geriatrics is the provision of optimal care for older adults with multiple chronic conditions, or 'multimorbidity'" (AGS, 2012b, p. 1957). Older adults experience normal age-related changes, such as those in pharmacokinetics and pharmacodynamics (Planton & Edlund, 2009), renal function (Bowling & O'Hare, 2012), and vision and hearing, and "often experience progressive decline in everyday function" (Lorenz et al., 2012, p. 468). They also age and live with a variety of disease-related chronic conditions such as diabetes (Germino, 2011; Ligthelm et al., 2012) and chronic kidney disease (Bowling & O'Hare, 2012; Campbell & O'Hare, 2008). Age-related changes and disease-related chronic conditions can significantly impact the lives of older adults, for example, by affecting the ability to ambulate; as previously mentioned, gait speed has been associated with life expectancy (Studenski et al., 2011).

Regardless of whether the chronic condition is a normal age-related change or the result of a disease process, older adults must adapt and live with these changes; in turn, providers and health care systems must learn to adapt and care for older adults living with multiple chronic conditions (AGS, 2012b). This adaptation should incorporate an understanding that disease-oriented approaches to care may not be the best approach for optimal care (Bowling and O'Hare, 2012; Tamura et al., 2012), and that deviation from clinical practice guidelines (Ligthelm et al., 2012; Maynard, O'Malley, & Kirsh, 2008) and specialized care units may be needed to deliver high-quality care.

The challenges of caring for older adults with multiple chronic conditions has led to the development of specialized care models designed to address their needs. The Acute Care for the Elderly (ACE) unit (Krall et al., 2012) is one model, while another is the Geriatric Resources for Assessment and Care of Elders (GRACE) (Bielaszka-DuVernay, 2011). The GRACE model is an integrated care model aimed at improving care for vulnerable elders who "suffer from a cluster of chronic conditions—for instance, hypertension, heart failure, and diabetes—and a large number contend with geriatric conditions such as depression, cognitive impairment, and physical limitations" (Bielaszka-DuVernay, p. 432).

The ACE unit and GRACE care model address older adults' chronic conditions at the system level, whereas the AGS's "Guiding Principles for the Care of Older Adults with Multimorbidity: An Approach for Clinicians" focuses on individual provider interactions and adaptations (2012a). This document recommends a number of strategies to improve the care of these patients, such as including them in decisions about treatment options when treatment for one condition may impact another condition. This strategy allows the patient to prioritize care based on personal preferences, cultural beliefs, and expectations. The health care system and providers need to emphasize using effective care strategies that prevent unnecessary adverse events and poor outcomes, as well as facilitate patient and caregiver involvement.

Increased Risk for Complications

The third attribute of individualized aging is older adults' increased risk for complications. This attribute is closely linked to the second attribute, age-related changes and multiple chronic conditions. Examples of potential risks older adults face include polypharmacy and suboptimal medication use (AGS, 2012a; Planton & Edlund, 2009), untreated or inadequate pain treatment (Curtiss, 2010); cancer (Balducci, Colloca, Cesari, & Gambassi, 2010), falls and falls with injury (Clyburn & Heydemann, 2011; Lakatos et al., 2009; Nitz et al., 2011), malnourishment (Feldblum, German, Castel, Harman-Boehm, & Shahar, 2011), microvascular complications and hypoglycemia (Germino, 2011; Ligthelm et al., 2012), hypotension (Maynard et al., 2008); iatrogenic complications (Krall et al., 2012), and complications from chronic kidney disease, such as cardiovascular events (Campbell & O'Hare, 2008).

Older adults are at increased risk for hypoglycemia, which can lead to "death and significant morbidity from seizures, comas, falls, fractures, and poor quality of life" (Ligthelm et al., 2012, p. 1565). Proper management of the risk for hypoglycemia can minimize the risk and decrease the possibility of adverse events. Similarly, adverse events from polypharmacy and suboptimal medication use, falls, diabetes and renal cardiovascular complications, iatrogenic complications, and a variety of other risk-related complications can be mitigated with skillful management by providers and a health care system that supports individualized care of older adults.

CONSEQUENCES

This analysis identified two consequences resulting from the concept of individualized aging: complexity of care over time and variable health outcomes. Consequences are contextual factors that occur as a result of the concept.

Complexity of Care Over Time

Aging is a process unique to each individual that occurs over time. As people age, their care becomes increasingly complex. Older adults are generally categorized in the health care literature as those individuals 65 years or older (Clyburn & Heydemann, 2011; Germino, 2011; Lewis, Griffith, Pignone, & Golin, 2009; Ligthelm et al., 2012; Wang et al., 2012). Yet older adults often live for decades past the age of 65. Over those ensuing decades, the aging process continues and is continually being influenced by personal experiences and biological processes. This leads to additional normal age-related changes and potentially to new or worsening chronic diseases. Episodic exacerbations of existing chronic diseases increase the complexity of an individual's care, as does the development of a new chronic disease, with the resultant potential for increasing the number of medications the person takes. As a person ages and develops more chronic diseases, additional medications are prescribed, leading to polypharmacy (administration of more than five medications) and complex medication regimens (Planton & Edlund, 2009).

Variable Health Outcomes

The second consequence of individualized aging is variable health outcomes. The heterogeneity of older adults, influenced by their past experiences and biological aging processes, contributes to variability in health outcomes. Variability in outcomes is also influenced by health care providers' ability to adapt to the unique needs of older adults, as well as older adults' interpretation of their health based on their past experiences, which influences how they access care and utilize support services and therefore significantly impacts their health outcomes.

An example of the complexity of the aging process (past experiences, biological decline, multiple chronic conditions, heterogeneity, and risk for complications) contributing to the variability of outcomes is visible in the use and application of clinical practice guidelines or protocols, which may lead to poor physiological and psychosocial outcomes if the unique heterogeneous needs and preferences of patients (AGS, 2012a) are not taken into consideration. Treatment strategies should be based on individualized plans of care that take into account the unique aspects of each older adult (Wang et al., 2012).

Two common diseases that are prevalent in the older adult population, diabetes (Germino, 2011; Ligthelm et al., 2012) and chronic renal disease (Bowling & O'Hare, 2012; Tamura et al., 2012) have well-established protocols, but those protocols may not be appropriate for every older adult. For example, the American Association of Clinical Endocrinologists recommends a hemoglobin A1c (HbA1c) of 6.5 percent or less for generally healthy adults (Handelsman et al., 2011), whereas the International Association of Gerontology and Geriatrics, the European Diabetes Working Party for Older People, and the International Task Force of Experts in Diabetes (Sinclair et al., 2012) recommend an HbA1c of between 7.0 and 7.5 percent for those over 70 years old.

Bowling and O'Hare (2012) contend that disease-oriented approaches to the care of older adults with chronic renal disease are not individualized enough to accommodate patients' comorbidities, preferences, and unique situations. Strict adherence to disease-oriented approaches may "carry more potential for harm than benefit if these [treatment strategies] fail to capture patient goals and preferences" (Bowling & O'Hare, p. 301). Some clinical practice guidelines may be appropriate—for example, the Beers criteria—but deviation from those guidelines may be appropriate after careful consideration of the individual older adult's needs, preferences, and comorbidities (Planton & Edlund, 2009). Others have examined the relationship of age to lung cancer treatment (Wang et al., 2012) and screening for colon cancer (Lewis et al., 2009) and recommended individualized treatments as the best approach for optimal outcomes.

Another reason for health care providers to consider deviation from or adaptation of clinical practice guidelines and protocols is the lack of older adults with multiple comorbidities enrolled in the studies that are used to develop the guidelines (AGS, 2012b; Campbell & O'Hare, 2008; Cheng & Nayar, 2009). Without older adults in the studies, their findings and recommendations may not support the best outcomes for these individuals.

Related Concepts

A related concept found in the literature was patient-centered care. Patient-centered care has been championed since the release of the IOM *Crossing the Quality Chasm* report (2001). Although patient-centered care is important to the overall quality of care, it is different from the concept of individualized aging. Patient-centered care focuses on ensuring that the health care system and providers focus on the needs of the patient and their family or caregivers and that providers not force care on patients, but rather collaborate with them on making care decisions based on the patients' personal beliefs, preferences, and desires. Individualized aging is a more granular concept that defines the process of aging from an individual perspective, but does not define how the health care system or providers should interact and collaborate with patients.

The concept of individualized aging provides additional knowledge of how patient-centered care should be delivered. Patient-centered care for older adults should encompass the attributes of individualized aging. For example, recognition that the older adult population is heterogeneous, lives with multiple chronic conditions, and is at risk for adverse events and complications if care is not individualized is essential to the delivery of high-quality care.

Definition of the Concept

Individualized aging is the complex interplay of past experiences and biological processes occurring within the heterogeneous population of older adults who live with multiple age-related changes and chronic conditions, putting them at risk for health care complications, adverse events, and poor outcomes. Individualized aging increases the complexity of care over time, which creates the potential for variable health outcomes that extends until death. Each older adult, due to unique circumstances related to his or her past experiences and biological aging processes, interprets and responds to aging in different ways, creating the full range of human responses to aging, chronic conditions, and risks for complications. On one end of the continuum are older adults with multiple chronic health conditions, limited social supports, and poor health outcomes, while at the other end are older adults with few chronic conditions, strong social supports, and good health outcomes. The range of possibilities along that continuum is as diverse as the older-adult population itself.

DISCUSSION

Individualized aging is an important concept for health care providers and students to understand. Past experiences and the psychological and sociological theories that help explain aging processes are important for shaping how older adults view the world around them. Essential to understanding the concept of individualized aging is recognition that the concept is not a measure or indicator of quality of life. Rather, the antecedents and attributes that define the concept provide the foundation for how each older adult interprets the aging process, thereby determining his or her overall quality of life. For example, cultural heterogeneity and past experiences affect how people live with and view age-related changes and chronic conditions, creating the range of human responses and experiences seen each day in health care settings. Each older adult's unique life experiences and interpretations of those experiences combine with their biological aging processes, interactions with the health care system, and availability of support services to influence their perception of their quality of life.

There are limitations to any concept analysis. This concept was structured around the health sciences literature, and therefore the antecedents, attributes, and consequences of individualized aging are connected to this particular context and time period. Also, the concepts of chronic disease and risk may evolve over time; therefore, future scholarly work should continue to define and clarify these concepts. Review of the literature in the humanities may have identified different attributes of aging, perhaps even sagacity. Future analyses of the concept from different contextual perspectives, such as from a humanities perspective, would broaden the understanding of the individual aging process.

CONCLUSION

This article defines a unique and important new concept to improve care of older adults: individualized aging. The antecedents of individualized aging—past experiences and biological aging processes—significantly impact older adults' lives and shape the core attributes of the concept. By focusing on the core attributes identified in this analysis—heterogeneity, living with age-related changes and chronic conditions, and increased risk for complications—health care providers will be able to improve the care of older adults. Recognition of the complexity of the care continuum will facilitate creation of systems that are proactive rather than reactive. Finally, rather than simply adhering to standardized guidelines and protocols that may not serve the patient's best interests, providers with an awareness of the core attributes of individualized aging will be able to make collaborative decisions with the patient, family, and other health care providers. Such decisions will be based on the unique needs and preferences of each older adult to achieve the optimal health outcomes.

*This scholarly project was funded by the Independence Foundation of Philadelphia.

References

Ahalt, C., Walter, L. C., Yourman, L., Eng, C., Pérez-Stable, E. J., & Smith, A. K. (2012). "Knowing is better": Preferences of diverse older adults for discussing prognosis. *Journal of General Internal Medicine, 27*(5), 568–575. doi:10.1007/s11606-011-1933-0

Almeida, O. P., Pirkis, J., Kerse, N., Sim, M., Flicker, L., Snowdon, J., . . . Pfaff, J. J. (2012). A randomized trial to reduce the prevalence of depression and self-harm behavior in older primary care patients. *Annals of Family Medicine, 10*(4), 347–356. doi:10.1370/afm.1368

American Association of Colleges of Nursing. (2010). *Recommended baccalaureate competencies and curricular guidelines for the nursing care of older adults: A supplement to the Essentials of Baccalaureate Education for Professional Nursing Practice.* Retrieved from www.aacn.nche.edu/geriatric-nursing/AACN_Gerocompetencies.pdf

American Geriatrics Society. (2012a). Guiding principles for the care of older adults with multimorbidity: An approach for clinicians. *Journal of the American Geriatrics Society, 60*, E1-E25. doi:10.1111/j.1532-5415.2012.04188.x

American Geriatrics Society. (2012b). Patient-centered care for older adults with multiple chronic conditions: A stepwise approach from the American Geriatrics Society. *Journal of the American Geriatrics Society, 60*, 1957–1968. doi:10.1111/j.1532-5415.2012.04187.x

Balducci, L., Colloca, G., Cesari, M., & Gambassi, G. (2010). Assessment and treatment of elderly patients with cancer. *Surgical Oncology, 19*(3), 117–123. doi:10.1016/j.suronc.2009.11.008

Berman, A., Mezey, M., Kobayashi, M., Fulmer, T., Stanley, J., Thornlow, D., & Rosenfeld, P. (2005). Gerontological nursing content in baccalaureate nursing programs: Comparison of findings from 1997 and 2003. *Journal of Professional Nursing, 21*(5), 268–275. doi:10.1016/j.profnurs.2005.07.005

Bielaszka-DuVernay, C. (2011). The "GRACE" model: In-home assessments lead to better care for dual eligibles. *Health Affairs, 30*(3), 431–434. doi:10.1377/hlthaff.2011.0043

Bowling, C. B., & O'Hare, A. M. (2012). Managing older adults with CKD: Individualized versus disease-based approaches. *American Journal of Kidney Disease, 59*(2), 293–302. doi:10.1053/j.ajkd.2011.08.039

Bradway, C., Trotta, R., Bixby, M. B., McPartland, E., Wollman, M. C., Kapustka, H., . . . Naylor, M. D. (2011). A qualitative analysis of an advanced practice nurse-directed transitional care model intervention. *Gerontologist, 52*(3), 394–407. doi:10.1093/geront/gnr078

Campbell, K. H., & O'Hare, A. M. (2008). Kidney disease in the elderly: Update on recent literature. *Current Opinions in Nephrology and Hypertension, 17*(3), 298–303. doi:10.1097/MNH.0b013e3282f5dd90

Cheng, J. W. M., & Nayar, M. (2009). A review of heart failure management in the elderly population. *American Journal of Geriatric Pharmacotherapy, 7*(5), 233–248. doi:10.1016/j.amjopharm.2009.10.001

Clyburn, T. A., & Heydemann, J. A. (2011). Fall prevention in the elderly: Analysis and comprehensive review of methods used in the hospital and in the home. *Journal of the American Academy of Orthopedic Surgeons, 19*(7), 402–409.

Cumming, E., & Henry, W. (1961). *Growing old: The process of disengagement.* New York, NY: Basic Books.

Curtiss, C. P. (2010). Challenges in pain assessment in cognitively intact and cognitively impaired older adults with cancer. *Oncology Nursing Forum, 37*(5), 7–16. doi:10.1188/10.ONF.S1.7-16

Eliopoulos, C. (2010). *Gerontological nursing* (7th ed.). Philadelphia, PA: Wolters Kluwer Health/Lippincott Williams & Wilkins.

Fabris, N. (1991). Neuroendocrine-immune interactions: A theoretical approach to aging. *Archives of Gerontology and Geriatrics, 12*, 219–230.

Feldblum, I., German, L., Castel, H., Harman-Boehm, I., & Shahar, D. R. (2011). Individualized nutritional intervention during and after hospitalization: The Nutrition Intervention Study clinical trial. *Journal of the American Geriatrics Society, 59*(1), 10–17. doi:10.1111/j.1532-5415.2010.03174.x

Franklin, P. D., Archbold, P. G., Fagin, C. M., Galik, E., Siegel, E., Sofaer, S., & Firminger, K. (2011). Building academic geriatric nursing capacity: Results after the first 10 years and implications for the future. *Nursing Outlook, 59*(4), 198–205. doi:10.1016/j.outlook. 2011.05.011

Germino, F. W. (2011). Noninsulin treatment of type 2 diabetes mellitus in geriatric patients: A review. *Clinical Therapeutics, 33*(12), 1868–1882. doi:10.1016/j.clinthera. 2011.10.020

Gilje, F., Lacey, L., & Moore, C. (2007). Gerontology and geriatric issues and trends in U.S. nursing programs: A national survey. *Journal of Professional Nursing, 23*(1), 21–29. doi:10.1016/j.profnurs.2006.12.001

Handelsman, Y., Mechanick, J. I., Blonde, L., Grunberger, G., Bloomgarden, Z. T., Bray, G. A., . . . Wyne, K. L. (2011). American Association of Clinical Endocrinologists medical guidelines for clinical practice for developing a diabetes mellitus comprehensive care plan. *Endocrine Practice, 17* (Suppl 2), 1–53. Retrieved from www.aace.com/files/dm-guidelines-ccp.pdf

Harman, D. (1956). Aging: A theory based on free radical and radiation chemistry. *Journal of Gerontology, 11*, 298–300.

Havighurst, R. J. (1961). Successful aging. *Gerontologist, 1*(1), 8–13. doi:10.1093/geront/1.1.8

Institute of Medicine. (2001). *Crossing the quality chasm: A new health system for the 21st century.* Washington, DC: National Academies Press.

Institute of Medicine. (2008). *Retooling for an aging America: Building the health care workforce.* Washington, DC: National Academies Press.

Institute of Medicine. (2011). *The future of nursing: Leading change, advancing health.* Washington, DC: National Academies Press.

Ironside, P. M., Tagliareni, M. E., McLaughlin, B., King, E., & Mengel, A. (2010). Fostering geriatrics in associate degree nursing education: An assessment of current curricula and clinical experiences. *Journal of Nursing Education, 49*(5), 246–252. doi:10.3928/01484834-20100217-01

Krall, E., Close, J., Parker, J., Sudak, M., Lampert, S., & Colonnelli, K. (2012). Innovation pilot study: Acute Care for the Elderly (ACE) unit – Promoting patient-centric care. *Health Environments Research and Design Journal, 5*(3), 90–98.

Lakatos, B. E., Capasso, V., Mitchell, M. T., Kilroy, S. M., Lussier-Cushing, M., Sumner, L., . . . Stern, T. A. (2009). Falls in the general hospital: Association with delirium, advanced age, and specific surgical procedures. *Psychosomatics, 50*(3), 218–226. doi:10.1176/appi.psy.50.3.218

Lewis, C. L., Griffith, J., Pignone, M. P., & Golin, C. (2009). Physicians' decisions about continuing or stopping colon cancer screening in the elderly: A qualitative study. *Journal of General Internal Medicine, 24*(7), 816–821. doi:10.1007/s11606-009-1006-9

Ligthelm, R. J., Kaiser, M., Vora, J., & Yale, J-F. (2012). Insulin in elderly adults: Risk of hypoglycemia and strategies for care. *Journal of the American Geriatrics Society, 60*(8), 1564–1570. doi:10.1111/j.1532-5415.2012.04055.x

Lorenz, R. A., Gooneratne, N., Cole, C. S., Kleban, M. H., Kalra, G. K., & Richards, K. C. (2012). Exercise and social activity improve everyday function in long-term care residents. *American Journal of Geriatric Psychiatry, 20*(6), 468–476. doi:10.1097/JGP.0b013e318246b807

Mänty, M., Heinonen, A., Leinonen, R., Törmäkangas, T., Hirvensalo, M., Kallienen, M., . . . Rantanen, T. (2009). Long-term effect of physical activity counseling on mobility limitation among older people: A randomized controlled study. *Journals of Gerontology: Series A, Biological Sciences and Medical Sciences, 64A*(1), 83–89. doi:10.1093/Gerona/gln029

Maulk, K. L. (2010). *Gerontological nursing: Competencies for care.* Sudbury, MA: Jones and Bartlett.

Maynard, G., O'Malley, C. W., & Kirsh, S. R. (2008). Perioperative care of the geriatric patient with diabetes or hyperglycemia. *Clinical Geriatric Medicine, 24*, 649–665. doi:10.1016/j.cger.2008.06.003

McCurry, S. M., LaFazia, D. M., Pike, K. C., Logsdon, R. G., & Teri, L. (2012). Development and evaluation of a sleep education program for older adults with dementia living in adult family homes. *American Journal of Geriatric Psychiatry, 20*(6), 494–504. doi:10.1097/JGP.0b013e318248ae79

Miller, C. A. (2012). *Nursing for wellness in older adults* (6th ed.). Philadelphia, PA: Wolters Kluwer Health/Lippincott Williams & Wilkins

National Council of State Boards of Nursing. (2008). *Consensus model for APRN regulation: Licensure, accreditation, certification & education.* Retrieved from www.ncsbn.org/Consensus_Model_for_APRN_Regulation_July_2008.pdf

The National League for Nursing. (2011). *Caring for older adults.* [National League for Nursing Vision Series]. Retrieved from www.nln.org/aboutnln/livingdocuments/pdf/nlnvision_2.pdf

Nitz, J., Cyarto, E., Andrews, S., Fearn, M., Fu, S., Haines, T., . . . Robinson, A. (2011). Outcomes from the implementation of facility-specific evidence-based falls prevention intervention program in residential aged care. *Geriatric Nursing, 31*(1), 41–50. doi:10.1016/j.gerinurse.2011.11.002

Parsons, J., Rouse, P., Robinson, E. M., Sheridan, N., & Connolly, M. J. (2012). Goal setting as a feature of homecare services for older people: Does it make a difference? *Age and Ageing, 41*, 24–29. doi:10.1093/ageing/afr118

Planton, J., & Edlund, B. J. (2009). Strategies for reducing polypharmacy in older adults. *Journal of Gerontological Nursing, 36*(1), 8–12.

Richards, C. K., Lambert, C., Beck, C. K., Bliwise, D. L., Evans, W. J., Gurpreet, K. K., . . . Sullivan, D. H. (2011). Strength training, walking, and social activity improve sleep in nursing home and assisted living residents: Randomized controlled trial. *Journal of the American Geriatrics Society, 59*(2), 214–223. doi:10.1111/j.1532-5415.2010.03246.x

Riley, M. W., Johnson, M., & Foner, A. (1972). *Aging and society: A sociology of age stratification* (Vol. 3). New York, NY: Russell Sage Foundation.

Rogers, B. L., & Knafl, K. A. (2000). *Concept development in nursing: Foundations, techniques, and applications* (2nd ed.). Philadelphia, PA: Saunders.

Sinclair, A., Morley, J. E., Rodriguez-Mañas, L., Paolisso, G., Bayer, T., Zeyfang, A., . . . Lorig, K. (2012). Diabetes mellitus in older people [Position statement on behalf of the International Association of Gerontology and Geriatrics (IAGG), the European Diabetes Working Party for Older People (EDWPOP), and the International Task Force of Experts in Diabetes]. *Journal of the American Medical Directors Association, 13*, 497–502. Retrieved from http://download.journals.elsevierhealth.com/pdfs/journals/1525-8610/PIIS1525861012001314.pdf

Studenski, S., Perera, S., Patel, K., Rosano, C., Faulkner, K., Inzitari, M., . . . Guralnik, J. (2011). Gait speed and survival in older adults. *Journal of the American Medical Association, 305*(1), 50–58. doi:10.1001/jama.2010.1923

Swain, S. L., & Nikolich-Zugich, J. (2009). Key research opportunities in immune system aging. *Journals of Gerontology: Series A, Biological Sciences and Medical Sciences 64A*(2), 183–186. doi:10.1093/gerona/gln068

Szanton, S. L., Thorpe, R. J., Boyd, C., Tanner, E. K., Leff, B., Agree, E., . . . Gitlin, L. N. (2011). Community aging in place, advancing better living for elders: A bio-behavioral-environmental intervention to improve function and health-related quality of life in disabled older adults. *Journal of the American Geriatrics Society, 59*(12), 2314–2320. doi:10.1111/j.1532-5415.2011.03698.x

Tagliareni, M. E., Cline, D. D., Mengel, A., McLaughlin, B., & King, E. (2012). Quality care for older adults: The NLN Advancing Care Excellence for Seniors (ACES) Project. *Nursing Education Perspectives, 33*(3), 144–149. doi:10.5480/1536-5026-33.3.144

Tamura, M. K., Tan, J. C., & O'Hare, A. M. (2012). Optimizing renal replacement therapy in older adults: A framework for making individualized decisions. *Kidney International, 82*, 261–269. doi:10.1038/ki.2011.384

Tjia, J., Givens, J. L., Karlawish, J. H., Okoli-Umeweni, A., & Barg, F. K. (2008). Beneath the surface: Discovering the unvoiced concerns of older adults with type 2 diabetes mellitus. *Health Education Research, 23*(1), 40–52. doi:10.1093/her/cyl161

Tornstam, L. (1994). Gerotranscendence: A theoretical and empirical exploration. In L. E. Thomas & S. A. Eisenhandler (Eds.). *Aging and the religious dimension* (pp. 203–225). Westport, CT: Auburn House.

Touhy, T. A., & Jett, K. F. (2012). *Ebersole and Hess' toward healthy aging: Human needs and nursing response* (8th ed.). St. Louis, MO: Elsevier.

Wang, S. Wong, M. L., Hamilton, N., Davoren, J. B., Jahan, T. M., & Walter, L. C. (2012). Impact of age and comorbidity on non-small-cell lung cancer treatment in older veterans. *Journal of Clinical Oncology, 30*(1), 1447–1455. doi:10.1200/JCO.2011.39.5269

3

Complexity of Care: A Concept Analysis of Older Adult Health Care Experiences

Daniel D. Cline, PhD, RN

ABSTRACT

PURPOSE: To define the term *complexity of care.*

BACKGROUND: The aging population and lack of gerontological preparation in pre-licensure nursing programs are pressing issues. The NLN Advancing Care Excellence for Seniors (ACE.S) project developed a framework to facilitate faculty and student understanding of older adults' care needs. Integral to the framework is the concept of complexity of care.

METHOD: Rogers and Knafl's evolutionary method of concept analysis was used.

RESULTS: The analysis identified three antecedents (focus on treatment and cure of disease, multiple comorbidities, and life experiences and culture), five attributes (polypharmacy, use of advanced technologies, novel care models, a fragmented health care system, and the relational nature of caregiving), and two consequences (impact on quality of life and impact on quality of care).

CONCLUSION: Defining the concept of complexity of care will facilitate student understanding of the unique health care needs of older adults.

By the year 2040 there will be an estimated 79.7 million older adults (those ages 65 years and older) living in the United States, approximately 14.1 million of whom will be 85 years old or older (U.S. Department of Health and Human Services [USDHHS], 2012). These older adults will be racially and ethnically diverse and live in a variety of care settings (e.g., home, assisted living community, long-term care). They will also be geographically diverse (urban and rural), have multiple chronic conditions, and take several prescription drugs and alternative and/or over-the-counter medications, all of which will contribute to frequent use of health care services (USDHHS).

The challenge the health care system and health care providers will face is how to provide high-quality care that succeeds in addressing the complex care needs of this population while also ensuring that older adults' well-being and quality of life are continually enhanced. This article focuses on defining the complex care issues older adults face so that pre-licensure nursing students will be better equipped to provide high-quality care when they enter the professional nurse workforce.

BACKGROUND

The seminal report *Retooling for an Aging America: Building the Health Care Workforce* (Institute of Medicine [IOM], 2008) highlights the serious lack of preparation and training the health care workforce currently receives in the specific care needs of older adults. This is true for the discipline of nursing (Ironside, Tagliareni, McLaughlin, King, & Mengel, 2010) as well as for other disciplines, such as medicine and dentistry (Bardach & Rowles, 2012).

The National League for Nursing (NLN) developed the Advancing Care Excellence for Seniors (ACE.S) project, as well as the ACE.S framework, in collaboration with the Community College of Philadelphia to provide a basis for nurse faculty to begin addressing the lack of gerontological education in pre-licensure nursing programs (Tagliareni, Cline, Mengel, McLaughlin, & King, 2012). Funding for development and dissemination of the NLN ACE.S Project was provided by the Independence Foundation, the John A. Hartford Foundation, and Laerdal Medical, and, since 2012, the Hearst Foundations.

The ACE.S project, which began in 2007, aims to improve the quality of care of older adults through innovations in education and faculty development and the fostering of gerontological nursing education in pre-licensure programs (NLN, 2013). It promotes gerontological nursing education by providing faculty with web resources, classroom-ready teaching tools and strategies, and faculty development seminars.

A key component of the project is the ACE.S framework, which is a conceptual tool that organizes important components of the project into a unifying whole. The framework provides faculty with a reference point from which to develop and teach the care of older adults. For students, the framework is a starting point for thinking about how to provide quality care to older adults. The ACE.S framework has three primary components: essential knowledge domains, essential nursing actions, and the learning environment, while its expected outcome is quality care for older adults.

The NLN ACE.S framework's essential knowledge domains are the unique concepts of individualized aging, complexity of care, and vulnerability during transitions. The definitions and descriptions of these concepts within the framework are unique and merit precision. Using concept analysis to define each domain will advance the ACE.S framework and improve gerontological nursing education by helping students better understand the unique health care needs of older adults. Concept analysis is essential to the advancement of nursing science (Rogers & Knafl, 2000), and further defining the three essential knowledge domains' core concepts will advance the use of the NLN ACE.S framework in nursing education research aimed at improving the care of older adults.

A concept is a mental image formed by synthesizing one's lived experiences, knowledge of phenomena, personal assumptions, and emotions. Concepts are abstractions and the building blocks of theories and conceptual frameworks (King & Fawcett, 1997). Theories and conceptual frameworks link concepts by using propositional statements to explain a particular phenomenon (King & Fawcett, 1997). Crucial to this process is consistency in the mental image held and in the understanding of a conceptual framework's concepts.

Because a concept is an abstract mental image, two individuals can have different mental images or understandings of the same concept. Therefore, analyses of concepts are necessary to clearly define and describe each concept used in a conceptual framework (Rogers & Knafl, 2000). Further, concept analyses provide definitions that are needed to operationalize concepts in frameworks, thus allowing researchers to test and use a framework to advance science and create new knowledge.

The NLN ACE.S framework concept of complexity of care is not clearly defined in the literature. The word *complex* is found throughout the health care literature and regularly used in describing the care needs of older adults. However, the vague and nonspecific use of the word *complex* or *complexity* does little to facilitate student learning and understanding of the complex care needs of older adults.

The Oxford Dictionary defines *complex* as "consisting of many different and connected parts; . . . not easy to analyze or understand; complicated or intricate" (Oxford Dictionaries, 2013). Although nursing students may understand the definition, their nascent care experiences limit their ability to understand the complexity involved in caring for older adults. A key challenge for nurse faculty and educators is facilitating that understanding.

The complexity-of-care concept is a core component of the NLN's ACE.S framework's essential knowledge domains. Therefore, the purpose of this analysis is to define *complexity of care* so as to provide a foundation from which students can interpret multifaceted clinical experiences with older adults. Doing so will also aid faculty by clarifying a rarely defined concept in teaching and discussing gerontological issues.

METHOD

The Rogers and Knafl (2000) evolutionary method of concept analysis was used for this analysis because of its focus on the contextual and temporal nature of concepts. Advancements in health care treatments and technologies, scientists' rapid decoding and understanding of human genetics, and society's evolving conceptualization of appropriate care for older adults support its use because future analyses may define *complexity of care* differently. The evolutionary method seeks to identify a set of attributes defining a concept so the concept can be identified in a variety of situations.

Sample

Literature relevant to the concept of complexity of care was identified in the nursing, medical, and social work literature. The bibliographic databases of CINAHL®, PubMed, and Web of Science™ were searched by combining the terms *complex* and *care* with each of the following: *aging, older adult, elderly,* and *geriatric.* The search was limited to the years 2007 (when the ACE.S project was launched) to 2013 and returned a total of 585 articles. Exclusion criteria included editorials, commentaries, conference abstracts and presentations, and reports of studies conducted outside the United States. Inclusion criteria included publication in an English-language, peer-reviewed journal. Review of each abstract for potential exclusion criteria and removal of duplicates reduced the number eligible for inclusion in the analysis to 173 articles. A random sample of 28, an adequate analytic sample size, was selected for the analysis.

Data Analysis

The analysis began by identifying how the word *complex* or *complexity* was used in each article. Because most articles did not provide a clear definition, an inductive process was used to identify the authors' intended meaning (Rogers & Knafl, 2000). It is important to recognize that the analysis presented in this article is based on the current use of *complex* or *complexity* in the health sciences literature.

FINDINGS

Analysis of the data revealed five attributes, three antecedents, and two consequences. These are connected to the definition of the concept; they are not factors that increase or decrease the care complexity. Therefore, attributes, for example, should not be seen as increasing complexity, but rather as factors that define the concept.

Antecedents

Antecedents are described by Rogers and Knafl (2000) as phenomena or events that occur prior to the concept of interest. They provide the context within which the attributes are interpreted. This analysis identified three antecedents of complexity of care: society's focus on treating and curing disease, multiple comorbidities, and life experiences and culture.

Focus on Treating and Curing Disease

The individual, systemic, and societal emphasis on treating and curing multiple diseases or disease processes was repeatedly found to be the focus of the articles reviewed. That focus plays a key role in the emergence of complex care. The attributes of complexity that were identified would not be relevant if there was no attempt to treat and cure disease. It is important to recognize that this antecedent does not imply that the individual or society should forgo treating and curing disease; rather, the desire to treat and cure disease is fundamental to creating much of the complexity seen with the care of older adults.

Multiple Comorbidities

The phenomenon of older adults living with multiple comorbidities is a relatively new one, which has arisen over the past half-century and contributes significantly to the attributes of complexity of care. The advances in technology, surgical interventions, and pharmacology result in people living longer and developing multiple comorbidities, which, in turn, create care complexity. Instead of dealing with one disease process, individuals, health care providers, and the health care system end up diagnosing, treating, and attempting to cure multiple disease processes, thereby creating conditions for complex care.

Past Experiences

Each person's life experiences affect how he or she interacts with health care providers, caregivers, and even the health care system as a whole. This can play a significant role in the degree of complexity.

Attributes

There are five attributes of complexity of care: polypharmacy, use of advanced technologies, novel care models, fragmentation of the health care system, and the relational nature of caregiving. The attributes only describe and define the aspects of the care that contribute to its complexity in older adults and do not confer a judgment on the appropriateness or ethical nature of that care. How complexity affects care and older adults' quality of life and well-being results in the consequences.

Polypharmacy

Polypharmacy is remarkably prevalent among older adults in the United States. It results from their multiple comorbidities and society's desire to treat these diseases using prescription medications. Medications are prescribed to treat symptoms, delay disease progression, and cure disease, and many older adults take several medications throughout the day (Barnason, Zimmerman, Hertzog, & Schulz, 2010; Elliott, 2012; McNabney et al., 2008; Moczygemba et al., 2011; Morrow et al., 2008; Page & Lindenfeld, 2012; Rhee, Csernansky, Emanuel, Chang, & Shega, 2011; Roth et al., 2008).

Polypharmacy contributes to complexity by creating situations where adherence to medication regimens cannot be achieved due to age-related cognitive and physical limitations affecting the ability to do so (Morrow et al., 2008; Roth et al., 2008), medication regimens being of such complexity that they are difficult to follow or understand (Barnason et al., 2010; Elliott, 2012; Morrow et al., 2008), and inadequate patient-provider communication that leads to confusion about the regimen (Barnason et al., 2010; Moczygemba et al., 2011). Polypharmacy also creates complexity due to poor communication during care transitions (Barnason et al., 2010), inappropriate prescribing (Elliott, 2012), and medication-related problems and interactions (Roth et al., 2008). Finally, polypharmacy creates financial challenges for older adults with limited income.

Use of Advanced Technologies

Advances in technologies and techniques to prolong the dying process have led to a significant number of older adults receiving complex care during the last few days of their lives, with as many as 80 percent receiving care in an intensive care unit (Ohta & Kronenfeld, 2011). But advanced technologies are not seen only in those circumstances. They also contribute to care complexity in the home setting as more and more older adults age in place at home. For example, in-home sensors are being developed and tested to monitor and provide audio prompts for patients with mild to moderate cognitive impairment (Bewernitz, Dasler, & Belchior, 2009). Such technologies have shown potential for improving self-care in persons with dementia, easing the burden on the caregiver by giving prompts and suggestions that cue appropriate activities and behaviors.

Technology also creates complexity in disease diagnosis. Emerging technologies are constantly improving diagnosis or identifying disease severity or progression. Innovation contributes to complexity because learning new procedures requires additional resources from the health care system, as well as from patients and families. Also, because emerging technologies are developed at the margins of scientific knowledge, they have the potential to increase the volume of diagnostic testing and of interventions that have limited impact on disease progression, but increase anxiety in older adults when tests are inconclusive or of limited clinical value (Illes, Rosen, Greicius, & Racine, 2007).

Novel Care Models

These emerge in response to older adults' multiple comorbidities, intricate medication regimens, and unique life circumstances. Transitional care models, an integral attribute of care complexity in older adults (Barnason et al., 2010; Nelson & Carrington, 2011; Ornstein, Smith, Foer, Lopez-Cantor, & Soriano, 2011), are often employed in coordinating transitions of patients with complex needs, particularly older adults with multiple comorbidities or functional or cognitive impairments (Nelson & Carrington, 2011).

Although transitional care models have been shown to improve patient outcomes (Barnason et al., 2010; Ornstein et al., 2011), they also increase care complexity. Successful models require the adoption of new roles by health care providers (particularly RNs and nurse practitioners), the education of patients and families about the role of the transitional care provider, and communication with and acceptance of the transitional care provider, among a host of other issues.

Novel care models also contribute to care complexity by introducing new roles and processes of care for health care professionals and patients. Some of the new models that have emerged focus on optimizing pharmacists to improve medication adherence and prevent avoidable medication-related health problems (Elliott, 2012; Moczygemba et al., 2011), having nurse practitioners telephone patients with diabetes to support their self-care (Amoako, Skelly, & Rossen, 2008), and conducting a shared medical appointment involving a group of patients with diabetes (Kirsh et al., 2007).

Unfamiliar methods such as these force older adults to accommodate a new way of interacting with health care providers (Kirsh et al., 2007). In addition, as the population of older adults grows, new models of care for use at assisted living facilities are emerging (McNabney et al., 2008). Other models recommend that nurse practitioners be allowed to serve as health care directors of nursing homes, creating parity with physicians, who are currently the only professionals the Center for Medicare and Medicaid Services allows to fill this role (Rogers, 2011).

Fragmented Health Care System

The inefficient and fragmented nature of the current US health care system contributes to the complexity of care by making communication among providers and between providers and patients difficult. This in turn can lead to medication errors or adverse events (Nelson & Carrington, 2011). The lack of cohesiveness leads to poor outcomes and provider frustration when acute care services are not closely coordinated with post-acute services (Ornstein et al., 2011), increasing the complexity of care.

Fragmentation also contributes to complexity by incentivizing providers and hospitals to improve the quality of care for some disease processes (e.g., infection rates) while potentially ignoring others (Snyder & Neubauer, 2007). Trends in health care reimbursement also contribute to complexity by incentivizing quality care for some disease processes (e.g., heart failure readmission) over others (Snyder & Neubauer, 2007). Other effects seen with fragmentation include potentially avoidable hospitalization (Walsh et al., 2012) and the frequent use of hospital emergency departments by older adults in nursing homes (Wang, Shah, Allman, & Kilgore, 2011). Hospitalizations or frequent visits to emergency departments due to inadequate discharge instructions or inappropriate ambulatory care resulting from a fragmented health care system also make older adults' care more complex.

Relational Nature of Caregiving

The care of older adults requires the interaction of two or more people, all or some of which may be between older adults and their family members or caregivers (Lingler, Sherwood, Crighton, Song, & Happ, 2008; Miller, Shoemaker, Willyard, & Addison, 2008; Rozario, Kidahashi, & DeRienzis, 2011), between older adults and their family members and health care providers (Judge, Menne, & Whitlatch, 2009; Sudore, Schillinger, Knight, & Fried, 2010; Torke et al., 2011; Utley-Smith et al., 2009), or between and among different types of health care providers (Anderson et al., 2012; Lekan, Hendrix, McConnell, & White, 2010; Toles & Anderson, 2011).

Interactions between older adults and their families often occur in connection with caregiving, as older adults begin to need assistance with managing everyday activities as a consequence of age-related changes or a disease process. Older adults may feel the need to express their independence in the face of diminishing functional ability by being reluctant or refusing to engage in activities suggested by a family member or caregiver. For example, Rozario et al. (2011) refer to "a recently widowed 78-year-old who lives in her own home [who said] in an interview, 'You know [my daughter] says, 'Do this.' . . . I tell her to leave me alone and I'm fine" (p. 230).

Rozario and colleagues (2011) also suggest that older adults may be reluctant to impose upon adult children or interfere in their lives. This can lead to complex care issues if the older adult needs assistance but is unwilling to use the available resources, such as a family member. Complexity of care can also be seen in the intricate balancing of the multiple tasks that caregivers must engage in to care for an older adult, producing caregiver stress (Miller et al., 2008) and a subsequent need to find ways to understand and cope with caregiver challenges.

Relationship dynamics between older adults and their families and health care providers also contribute to care complexity. Whether those interactions are staff interactions with family and older adults recently admitted to a nursing home (Utley-Smith et al., 2009) or discussions of end-of-life care with surrogate decision makers in the intensive care unit of a hospital (Torke et al., 2011), the way in which the health care provider, the older adult, and the latter's family view and understand the situation is crucial in determining the complexity of the situation. For example, Sudore and colleagues (2010) found that older adults who are racial and ethnic minorities and those with limited health literacy faced more decisional uncertainty when asked about advanced care decisions, such as being put on or forgoing life support.

If providers fail to account for the older adult's perspective on and understanding of a situation based on his or her life experiences and cultural background, the differing expectations of the provider and the older adult make care more complex. Judge and colleagues (2009) also suggest that providers caring for patients with dementia should understand the stressors and care needs of their patients for effective communication and best outcomes to occur. Finally, complexity of care is also influenced by the relational aspect of health care providers interacting among themselves, whether that is through the implementation of new evidence-based guidelines (Anderson et al., 2012; Lekan et al., 2010) or the management practices of clinical supervisors (Toles & Anderson, 2011).

Consequences

This analysis identified two consequences of the concept of complexity of care: impact on quality of life and impact on quality of care. Consequences are events or phenomena that occur after the concept of interest and are a result of its attributes. Each attribute may contribute to both of the consequences.

Impact on Quality of Life

The attributes identified for complexity of care can have a significant impact on an older adult's quality of life, one that is either positive or negative depending on how the complexity is managed. For example, older adults with multiple comorbidities require polypharmacy (McNabney et al., 2008). The medications they take on a daily basis are important for treating and managing their multiple chronic diseases. When prescribed and taken appropriately, older adults with complex polypharmacy challenges can mitigate the diseases' potential adverse health effects. However, poorly managed polypharmacy can lead to a poor quality of life if it necessitates repeated hospital admissions or causes other adverse events (Moczygemba et al., 2011).

Impact on Quality of Care

Poorly managed polypharmacy can also create the second consequence of complexity of care. Adverse health events or hospitalization represent poor quality of care management because these events could have been prevented.

The positive and negative consequences of care complexity can be seen through a variety of the attributes. For example, advanced technologies provide opportunities for early diagnosis or better understanding of disease progression, which could improve quality of life; conversely, when treatment options are not available, better diagnostic technologies may diminish quality of life by adding stress and uncertainty to an older adult's life. Novel care models such as shared medical appointments (Kirsh et al., 2007) can significantly improve an older adult's clinical disease process, thus impacting quality of care, while also impacting quality of life by preventing disease-related complications.

Definition of the Concept

Complexity of care is defined as a focus on simultaneously treating and curing multiple disease processes, which leads to polypharmacy, use of advanced technologies, and the creation of novel care models. The concept is further defined by a fragmented health care system and the relational nature of caregiving. Complexity of care directly affects older adults by having positive or negative impacts on their quality of life and the quality of the care they receive.

DISCUSSION

Nurse educators must begin adapting to the rapidly growing older adult population by incorporating specific content connected with the care of older adults into their courses; geriatric content should be included in educational curricula from pre-licensure through master's and doctoral education. To facilitate this fusion, the NLN ACE.S project aims to supply nursing faculty with the tools and resources needed to effectively incorporate gerontological content into pre-licensure nursing programs' classroom, clinical, laboratory, and simulation settings. Doing so effectively requires having an understanding of what key principles should be incorporated. The ACE.S conceptual framework identifies several of these key principles, including the topic of this paper, complexity of care.

Complexity of care is an essential concept for health care providers—especially nurses—to understand. Older adult care is complex, but simply stating this to students with limited clinical experience does little to help them understand the concept. Educators must be able to define what is meant by *complexity* in order for students to understand the implications and the ways in which complexity can improve as well as diminish an older adult's life. Most importantly, nursing students need to recognize that complexity itself is neither bad nor good; rather, what is important is to *manage* complexity. Many older adults choose to treat their chronic diseases. This can lead to polypharmacy, the use of advanced technologies, and the development of new models of care. When these realities intersect with our fragmented health care system and an individual's expectations and past experiences, those individuals' care becomes complex.

Nurses and other health care providers need to focus on managing complexity, rather than on decreasing it. As life expectancy continues to rise and advances in treatments and technologies further lengthen life, people will also develop more chronic disease. Complexity needs to be managed and recognized as offering the potential to significantly improve older adults' quality of life and of care.

Two important resources available through the NLN ACE.S Project can be utilized by faculty in teaching complexity of care to pre-licensure students: the NLN ACE.S unfolding cases and a series of teaching strategies. The unfolding cases are designed to provide students with a holistic understanding of older adults. The stories they contain unfold over time and are designed for use in simulation experiences. The teaching strategies are a series of teaching/learning activities that have been used by educators to engage students in learning about complex care issues facing older adults. (Both resources can be found at www.nln.org/ACES.)

This analysis, like all analyses, had limitations. The data used came from the health sciences literature covering a specific time period. Therefore, analyses that incorporate different sources of data—for example, those reviewing humanities literature—may identify different antecedents, attributes, and consequences of the concept of complexity of care. In addition, the evolutionary method of concept analysis used for this analysis has a temporal dimension, and a similar analysis done in the future will likely identify different attributes of complexity depending on how society and technology evolve. Because health care changes at such a rapid pace, the concept of complexity of care should be re-explored as it evolves over time.

CONCLUSION

This article defines the unique concept of complexity in caring for older adults. The antecedents of this concept—a focus on treating and curing disease, multiple comorbidities, and an individual's life experiences and culture—impact the attributes of polypharmacy, advanced care technologies, novel care models, a fragmented health care system, and the relational nature of caregiving. New nurses who enter the health care system with an understanding of what care complexity means and entails for older adults will be better prepared to manage that complexity, leading to better care and outcomes.

The nursing profession must be a leader in the effort to increase the amount and quality of gerontological content in pre-licensure health care programs. However, nursing must also be at the forefront of improving care to older adults by advancing theories and approaches like the ACE.S framework that define important constructs of the care of older adults. Theoretical work such as concept analyses will benefit student learning and research by defining important concepts of caring for older adults.

*This scholarly project was funded by the Independence Foundation of Philadelphia.

References

Amoako, E., Skelly, A. H., & Rossen, E. K. (2008). Outcomes of an intervention to reduce uncertainty among African American women with diabetes, *Western Journal of Nursing Research, 30*(8), 928–942. doi:10.1177/0193945908320465

Anderson, R. A., Corazzini, K., Porter, K., Daily, K., McDaniel, R. R., & Colón-Emeric, C. (2012). CONNECT for quality: Protocol of a cluster randomized controlled trial to improve fall prevention in nursing homes. *Implementation Science, 7*(11), 1–14.

Bardach, S. H., & Rowles, G. D. (2012). Geriatric education in the health professions: Are we making progress? *Gerontologist, 52*(5), 607–618.

Barnason, S., Zimmerman, L., Hertzog, M., & Schulz, P. (2010). Pilot testing of a medication self-management transition intervention for heart failure patients. *Western Journal of Nursing Research, 32*(7), 849–870. doi:10.1177/0193945910371216

Bewernitz, M. W., Dasler, M. A., & Belchior, P. (2009). Feasibility of machine-based prompting to assist persons with dementia. *Assistive Technology, 21*, 196–207. doi:10.1080/10400430903246050

Elliott, R. A. (2012). Reducing medication regimen complexity for older patients prior to discharge from hospital: Feasibility and barriers. *Journal of Clinical Pharmacy Therapeutics, 37*(6), 637–642. doi:10.1111/j.1365–2710.2012.01356.x

Illes, J., Rosen, A., Greicius, M., & Racine, E. (2007). Prospects for prediction: Ethics analysis of neuroimaging in Alzheimer's disease. *Annals of the New York Academy of Sciences, 1097*, 278–295. doi:10.1196/annals.1379.030

Institute of Medicine. (2008). *Retooling for an aging America: Building the health care workforce.* Washington, DC: National Academies Press.

Ironside, P. M., Tagliareni, M. E., McLaughlin, B., King, E., & Mengel, A. (2010). Fostering geriatrics in associate degree nursing education: An assessment of current curricula and clinical experiences. *Journal of Nursing Education, 49*(5), 246–252. doi:10.3928/01484834–20100217–01

Judge, K. S., Menne, H. L., & Whitlatch, C. J. (2009). Stress process model for individuals with dementia. *Gerontologist, 50*(3), 294–302. doi:10.1093/geront/gnp162

King, I. M., & Fawcett, J. (1997). *The language of nursing theory and metatheory.* Indianapolis, IN: Center Nursing Publishing.

Kirsh, S., Watts, S., Pascuzzi, K., O'Day, M. E., Davidson, D., Strauss, G., . . . Aron, D. C. (2007). Shared medical appointments based on the chronic care model: A quality improvement project to address the challenges of patients with diabetes with high cardiovascular risk. *BMJ Quality and Safety in Health Care, 16*, 349–353. doi:10.1136/qshc.2006.019158

Lekan, D., Hendrix, C. C., McConnell, E. S., & White, H. (2010). The connected learning model for disseminating evidence-based care practices in clinical settings. *Nurse Education in Practice, 10*, 243–248. doi:10.1016/j.nepr.2009.11.013

Lingler, J. H., Sherwood, P. R., Crighton, M. H., Song, M.-K., & Happ, M. B. (2008). Conceptual challenges in the study of caregiver-care recipient relationships. *Nursing Research, 57*(5), 367–372. doi:10.1097/01.NNR.0000313499.99851.0c

McNabney, M. K., Samus, Q. M., Lyketsos, C. G., Brandt, J., Onyike, C. U., Baker, A., & Rosenblatt, A. (2008). The spectrum of medical illness and medication use among residents of assisted living facilities in central Maryland. *Journal of the American Medical Directors Association, 9*(8), 558–564. doi:10.1016/j.jamda.2008.03.003

Miller, K. I., Shoemaker, M. M., Willyard, J., & Addison, P. (2008). Providing care for elderly parents: A structural approach to family caregiver identity. *Journal of Family Communication, 8*, 19–43. doi:10.1080/15267430701389947

Moczygemba, L. R., Barner, J. C., Lawson, K. A., Brown, C. M., Gabrillo, E. R., Godley, P., & Johnsrud, M. (2011). Impact of telephone medication therapy management on medication and health-related problems, medication adherence, and Medicare Part D drug costs: A 6-month follow up. *American Journal of Geriatric Pharmacotherapy, 9*(5), 328–338. doi:10.1016/j.amjopharm.2011.08.001

Morrow, D., Raquel, L., Schriver, A., Redenbo, S., Rozovski, D., & Weiss, G. (2008). External support for collaborative problem solving in a simulated provider/patient medication scheduling task. *Journal of Experimental Psychology Application, 14*(3), 288–297. doi:10.1037/a0012809

The National League for Nursing. (2013). Faculty resources: ACES Advancing Care Excellence for Seniors. Retrieved from www.nln.org/facultyprograms/facultyresources/aces/index.htm

Nelson, J. N., & Carrington, J. M. (2011). Transitioning the older adult in the ambulatory care setting. *Association of Operating Room Nurses Journal, 94*(4), 348–358. doi:10.1016/j.aorn.2011.04.025

Ohta, B., & Kronenfeld, J. J. (2011). Intensity of acute care services at the end of life: Nonclinical determinants of treatment variation in an older adult population. *Journal of Palliative Medicine, 14*(6), 722–728. doi:10.1089/jpm.2010.0360

Ornstein, K., Smith, K. L., Foer, D. H., Lopez-Cantor, M. T., & Soriano, T. (2011). To the hospital and back home again: A nurse practitioner-based transitional care program for hospitalized homebound people. *Journal of the American Geriatrics Society, 59*(3), 544–551. doi:10.1111/j.1532-5415.2010.03308.x

Oxford Dictionaries. (2013). Complex. *Oxford Dictionaries Online.* Retrieved from www.oxforddictionaries.com/us/definition/american_english/complex?q=complex

Page, R. L., & Lindenfeld, J. (2012). The comorbidity conundrum: A focus on the role of noncardiovascular chronic conditions in the heart failure patient. *Current Cardiology Reports, 14*(3), 276–284. doi:10.1007/s11886-012-0259-9

Rhee, Y., Csernansky, J. G., Emanuel, L. L., Chang, C. G., & Shega, J. W. (2011). Psychotropic medication burden and factors associated with antipsychotic use: An analysis of a population-based sample of community-dwelling older persons with dementia. *Journal of the American Geriatric Society, 59*(11), 2100–2107. doi:10.1111/j.1532-5415.2011.03660.x

Rogers, B. L., & Knafl, K. A. (2000). *Concept development in nursing: Foundations, techniques, and applications* (2nd ed.). Philadelphia, PA: Saunders.

Rogers, G. (2011). Gerontological NPs as healthcare directors of nursing homes. *Journal for Nurse Practitioners, 7*(2), 132–135.

Roth, M. T., Moore, C. G., Ivey, J. L., Esserman, D. A., Campbell, W. H., & Weinberger, M. (2008). The quality of medication use in older adults: Methods of a longitudinal study. *American Journal of Geriatric Pharmacotherapy, 6*(4), 220–233. doi:10.1016/j.amjopharm.2008.10.004

Rozario, P. A., Kidahashi, M., & DeRienzis, D. R. (2011). Selection, optimization, and compensation: Strategies to maintain, maximize, and generate resources in later life in the face of chronic illness. *Journal of Gerontological Social Work, 54*, 224–239. doi:10.1080/01634372.2010.539589

Snyder, L., & Neubauer, R. L. (2007). Pay-for-performance principles that promote patient-centered care: An ethics manifesto. *Annals of Internal Medicine, 147*(11), 792–794.

Sudore, R. L., Schillinger, D., Knight, S. J., & Fried, T. R. (2010). Uncertainty about advanced care planning treatment preferences among diverse older adults. *Journal of Health Communications, 15*, 159–171. doi:10.1080/108110730.2010.499982

Tagliareni, M. E., Cline, D. D., Mengel, A., McLaughlin, B., & King, E. (2012). Quality care for older adults: The NLN Advancing Care Excellence for Seniors (ACES) Project. *Nursing Education Perspectives, 33*(3), 144–149. doi:10.5480/1536–5026–33.3.144

Toles, M., & Anderson, R. A. (2011). State of the science: Relationship-oriented management practices in nursing homes. *Nursing Outlook, 59*, 221–227. doi:10.1016/j.outlook.2011.05.001

Torke, A. M., Sachs, G. A., Helft, P. R., Petronio, S., Purnell, C., Hui, S., & Callahan, C. M. (2011). Timing of do-not-resuscitate orders for hospitalized older adults who require a surrogate decision maker. *Journal of the American Geriatrics Society, 59*, 1326–1331. doi:10.1111/j.1532–5415.2011.03480.x

U.S. Department of Health and Human Services, Administration for Community Living, Administration on Aging. (2012). *A profile of older Americans: 2012.* Retrieved from www.aoa.gov/Aging_Statistics/Profile/2012/docs/2012profile.pdf

Utley-Smith, Q., Colón-Emeric, C. S., Lekan-Rutledge, D., Ammarell, N., Bailey, D., Corazzini, K., . . . Anderson, R. A. (2009). Staff perceptions of staff-family interactions in nursing homes. *Journal of Aging Studies, 23*(3), 168–177. doi:10.1016/j.jaging.2007.11.003

Walsh, E. G., Wiener, J. M., Haber, S., Bragg, A., Freiman, M., & Ouslander, J. G. (2012). Potentially avoidable hospitalizations of dually eligible Medicare and Medicaid beneficiaries from nursing facilities and home and community-based services waiver programs. *Journal of the American Geriatrics Society, 60*, 821–829. doi:10.1111/j.1532–5415.2012.03920.x

Wang, H. E., Shah, M. N., Allman, R. M., & Kilgore, M. (2011). Emergency department visits by nursing home residents in the United States. *Journal of the American Geriatrics Society, 59*, 1864–1872. doi:10.1111/j.1532–5415.2011.03587.x

4

A Concept Analysis of Vulnerability During Transitions

Daniel D. Cline, PhD, RN

ABSTRACT

AIM: Define the concept of *vulnerability during transitions*.

BACKGROUND: There is a need to produce RNs with the knowledge, skills, and attitudes (KSAs) necessary to care for the increasing older adult population. The NLN Advancing Care Excellence for Seniors (ACE.S) project developed a framework to help faculty and pre-licensure students develop these KSAs. Key to this framework is the concept of vulnerability during transitions.

METHOD: Rogers and Knafl's evolutionary method of concept analysis.

RESULTS: The analysis revealed two antecedents (use of multiple medications to treat disease, fragmentation of the health care system), two attributes (inadequate continuity of care; poor communication and coordination of care among health care providers, patients, and families), and two consequences (readmission to a previous or new care setting, potential negative health outcomes).

CONCLUSION: Knowledge of the antecedents, attributes, and consequences of vulnerability during transitions will facilitate improved care for older adults in all settings.

As members of the "baby boom" generation increase their access to and utilization of health care services, nurses, physicians, pharmacists, and other providers will require specialized knowledge, skills, and attitudes (KSAs) to address their health care needs. However, there is a shortage of health care professionals, nurses in particular, who are trained and educated to care for the growing population of persons over 65 years of age (Berman et al., 2005; Gilje, Lacey, & Moore, 2007; Institute of Medicine [IOM], 2008; Ironside, Tagliareni, McLaughlin, King, & Mengel, 2010).

BACKGROUND

The lack of gerontological nursing content in both baccalaureate and associate degree programs has been well described (Gilje, Lacey, & Moore, 2007; Ironside et al., 2010). A key factor in the failure to teach gerontological nursing content in pre-licensure nursing programs is the shortage of faculty with gerontological expertise, training, and experience who are competent to design and lead curricular revisions that are inclusive of care principles for older adults (Latimer & Thronlow, 2006). Faculty who are qualified to teach these courses are also needed by pre-licensure programs.

As the health care system evolves in response to financial and system-level constraints, older adults will find themselves experiencing multiple transitions across a variety of health care settings. Therefore, it is important that faculty be well versed in this specific area of gerontological knowledge. Faculty need to understand how transitions across and within health care settings, as well as within an older adult's life (e.g., loss of a spouse), impact health and well-being. This understanding will be crucial for ensuring the delivery of high-quality care to older adults; transferring this knowledge to novice nurses should be an important part of all pre-licensure programs.

Over the past several years, nursing organizations and philanthropic foundations have developed a number of strategies and initiatives to ensure that our future nursing workforce is prepared for the specialized care of older adults. Two organizations that have led efforts to address gerontological nursing content deficiencies in pre-licensure programs are the National League for Nursing (NLN) and the American Association of Colleges of Nursing (AACN). A major initiative developed by the AACN, in partnership with the John A. Hartford Foundation (JAHF), was the creation and publication of the *Baccalaureate Competencies for Nursing Care of Older Adults* (AACN, 2010), designed to enhance the AACN *Essentials of Baccalaureate Education for Professional Nursing Practice* (2008). This publication provides an impressive list of competencies and serves as an excellent roadmap of the KSAs nurses should have upon graduation. The competencies lace the ability to provide faculty with a deeper understanding of the specialized needs and circumstances that surround the care of older adults.

The NLN centered its efforts to enhance gerontological nursing in pre-licensure nursing programs through the development of the Advancing Care Excellence for Seniors (ACE.S) project (www.nln.org/aces). The ACE.S project, developed in collaboration with the Community College of Philadelphia and funded by the Independence Foundation, the JAHF, Laerdal Medical, and, since 2012, the Hearst Foundations, enhances gerontological nursing content in pre-licensure programs through the development of the NLN ACE.S framework (Tagliareni, Cline, Mengel, McLaughlin, & King, 2012) and content enrichment. Some of the educational enrichments the ACE.S program promotes are online resources for faculty and students, classroom-ready teaching tools and strategies, and unfolding case studies and simulations that target specific gerontological care needs.

The NLN ACE.S framework provides a model for teaching and learning the care of older adults (Tagliareni et al., 2012). It has three key components: Essential Knowledge Domains, Essential Nursing Actions, and the Learning Environment. The knowledge domains and the essential nursing actions interact synergistically within the learning environment, thereby contributing to and enhancing student KSAs about older adults.

Within the knowledge domains component are three unique concepts: *individualized aging, complexity of care,* and *vulnerability during transitions.* In order to advance understanding of the NLN ACE.S framework and enhance pre-licensure gerontological nursing content, these three concepts must be defined and described. The concepts of individualized aging and complexity of care have been described previously (Cline, 2014, 2015).

The purpose of this concept analysis is to define and clarify the NLN ACE.S framework concept of *vulnerability during transitions.* The Merriam-Webster (2015) dictionary definition of *vulnerability* is: "capable of being easily hurt or harmed physically, mentally, or emotionally"; *transitions* is defined as "a change from one state or condition to another." Previous works on the conceptualization of vulnerability have identified the need to conceptualize vulnerability in the context of society, communities, economics, race, gender, and class (Tomm-Bonde, 2012). Vulnerability as a concept has also been described as highly individualized, leaving a person open to positive or negative health outcomes (Purdy, 2004). This article explores the concept for older adults who experience transitions.

METHOD

The evolutionary method of concept analysis (Rogers & Knafl, 2000) was used for this study as it focuses on the concept's contextual and temporal nature. Concept analysis aims to identify a set of attributes that "constitute a real definition" (Rogers & Knafl, p. 91), so that it is possible to characterize situations or experiences that encompass the concept. It also provides a basis for further research on the concept as antecedents, attributes, and consequences are inclined to change and evolve over time.

Sample

Literature relevant to the concept of vulnerability during transitions was identified in the health sciences literature. The following search terms were used to search the PubMed and Web of Science bibliographic databases: vulnerability AND transitions AND (a) older adults, (b) elderly, and (c) geriatric. The search was limited to articles in the English language, sample ages greater than or equal to 65, and published dates between 2007 and 2013. This search, which produced 191 studies, was followed by a review of the article abstracts. Articles were excluded if they were conference presentations or conducted outside the United States. Articles were also excluded if they did not relate to the concept of vulnerability during transitions (e.g., articles on transitions between rapid eye movement [REM] sleep and non-REM sleep in older adults). This left a final sample of 85 articles for review. Of the remaining 85 articles, 26 articles (30 percent) were randomly sampled for use in this review. The Rodgers and Knafl method recommends that at least 20 percent of the sample be used in the analysis.

Data Analysis

Each article was reviewed to understand how the concept of vulnerability during transitions was used. Most articles did not clearly define vulnerabilities during transitions; however, according to Rogers and Knafl (2000), this is not uncommon. Therefore, inductive reasoning was used to examine how authors used or presented the concept. Specific data elements were extracted into a table to organize the data and get a sense of how the concept was being used.

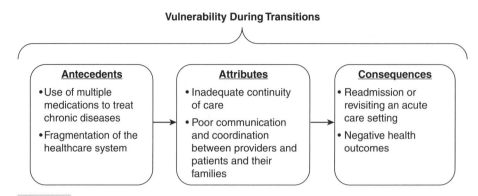

FIGURE 4.1 Antecedents, attributes, and consequences of vulnerability during transitions.

FINDINGS

Analysis of the data revealed two antecedents, two defining attributes, and two conse-quences. (See Figure 4.1.) Examples of specific textual data from the sample are used to describe them.

Antecedents

Antecedents are those events that occur prior to the concept of interest (Rogers & Knafl, 2000). This analysis identified two antecedents for the concept of vulnerability during transitions: (1) use of multiple medications to treat disease, and (2) fragmentation of the health care system.

Use of Multiple Medications

The use of multiple medications is a key antecedent that contributes to vulnerabil-ity during transitions for older adults. A critical aspect of this antecedent is the lack of clear processes to accurately describe and provide detailed information about an older adult's medication regime between transitions in care settings (Foust, Naylor, Bixby, & Ratcliffe, 2012; Gleason et al., 2010; Hu, Capezuti, Foust, Boltz, & Kim, 2012; Rose et al., 2013; Toles, Barroso, Colon-Emeric, Corazzini, McConnell, & Anderson, 2012). This issue can be further com-plicated when older adults take large numbers of medications (Gleason et al., 2010), when cultural and language barrier challenges are present (Hu et al., 2012), or when there is required monitoring of therapeutic levels (Rose et al., 2013).

Fragmentation of the Health Care System

A second antecedent that contributes to the concept is the fragmentation of the United States health care system. Gaps in care and the fragmentation of the health care sys-tem contribute to vulnerability as they create periods of uncertainty for older adults. For example, older adults are likely to lose their dental health care coverage upon entering retirement, which may contribute to irregular visits to dental health care practitioners

(Manski et al., 2011). Dental care is not covered by Medicare, and there is low likelihood of obtaining dental insurance after retirement (Manski et al., 2009). Research has indicated significant associations between oral health and systemic health. This aspect of health care fragmentation contributes to the vulnerability of older adults and is normally not considered by practitioners. To identify gaps in care, practitioners should consider the full range of health care services older adults should be able to access.

Fragmentation of care at the end of life also contributes to vulnerability (Teno et al., 2013). It contributes also to the high utilization of intensive care services and the low utilization of hospice. Teno et al. reported that older adults had three or more hospitalizations in the last 90 days of life and used hospice for three days or less before death.

Fragmentation of care is also seen in the new Affordable Care Act (Naylor et al., 2012), which focuses many innovations on the acute care needs of older adults and excludes older adults in long-term care. Provisions in the law attempt to improve care for specific diseases by incentivizing hospitals to prevent readmissions; however, the complex and multifactorial nature of geriatric syndromes means that hospitals may overlook or ignore the complexity of an older adult's health to focus on a single disease. The new law seems to do little to extend incentives for quality care beyond the acute-care episode (Naylor et al., 2012). These fragmentations create vulnerabilities for older adults as they move and transition from one setting to the next or from one life event to the next.

Attributes

The two overarching attributes of vulnerability during transitions are: (1) inadequate continuity of care and (2) poor communication and coordination of care among health care providers and patients and their families.

Inadequate Continuity of Care

McNabney et al. (2009) aptly state that providers should develop the ability to guide patients and families through various care models across the continuum of care accessed by older adults, thereby ensuring continuity of care. Unfortunately, providers often do not have this ability, which becomes a defining feature of the vulnerability of older adults. Continuity of care between outpatient and inpatient settings can reduce the odds of having an intensive care admission during a terminal hospitalization (Sharma, Freeman, Zhang, & Goodwin, 2009), decreasing the likelihood of death taking place in the high-technology and impersonal critical-care environment.

For patients with dementia, the failure to have continuity of care during multiple transitions can lead to medical errors, miscommunication, and care that conflicts with the wishes of the patient and family (Callahan et al., 2010). When care providers are well acquainted with typical disease and care transitions for patients and family members dealing with dementia, they can facilitate transitions and the continuity of care by providing guidance and ensuring that the right level of care is provided (Rose & Palan Lopez, 2012). Several studies have shown that continuity failures between emergency-care settings and home- and long-term-care settings also contribute to vulnerabilities during transitions (Boltz, Parke, Shuluk, Capezuti, & Galvin, 2012; Terrell et al., 2009; Vashi et al., 2013).

Poor Coordination of Care and Communication Among Health Care Providers, Patients, and Families

Failures of communication and coordination are core attributes of older adult vulnerabilities during transitions (Arora et al., 2010; Boxer et al., 2012; Enguidanos, Gibbs, & Jamison, 2012; Nahm, Resnick, Orwig, Magaziner, & DeGrezia, 2010; Parrish, O'Malley, Adams, Adams, & Coleman, 2009; Parry, Min, Chugh, Chalmers, & Coleman, 2009; Shippee, 2009; Toles, Barroso, Colon-Emeric, Corazzini, McConnell, & Anderson, 2012; Takahashi et al., 2013). When a patient transitions from the hospital setting to another health care setting, coordination and communication among providers and patients is crucial to preventing adverse outcomes. Arora et al. (2010) found that patients identified problems or delays obtaining follow-up tests, appointments, or test results, and that patients were also readmitted to the hospital or emergency department for necessary reevaluations.

When processes are in place to facilitate transitions, either by nurse practitioners (Enguidanos et al., 2012; Takahashi, et al., 2013), registered nurses (Parry et al., 2009), primary care physicians (Arora et al., 2010), or others such as social workers or trained community workers (Parrish et al., 2009), older adults are less vulnerable. Coordination and communication among providers and patients during transitions can lead to fewer emergency department visits, fewer rehospitalizations, and improved perceived health status in the older adult experiencing the transition (Dedhia et al., 2009). This is also true for older adults in other settings. Boxer et al. (2012) found communication and coordination to be crucial to preventing high recidivism rates for heart failure patients discharged from hospitals to nursing homes.

In a study that examined older adults' transitions within a comprehensive care facility that contained independent living, assisted living, and long-term nursing care options, communication and coordination also contributed to vulnerability during transitions between levels of care (e.g., independent living to assisted living) (Shippee, 2009). Communication and coordination were crucial to mitigating feelings of social disengagement and feelings of disempowerment.

Consequences

Consequences are contextual factors that occur as a result of the concept. This analysis identified two consequences related to the concept of vulnerability during transitions: (1) readmission to a previous or new care setting, and (2) potential negative health outcomes.

Readmission to a Previous or New Care Setting

Major consequences of the concept's attributes of inadequate continuity of care and poor communication and coordination are readmissions to previous or new care settings (Dedhia, et al., 2009; Foust, Naylor, Bixby, & Ratcliffe, 2012; Gill, Allore, Gahbauer, & Murphy, 2010; Gleason, et al., Hu, Capezuti, Foust, Boltz, & Kim, 2012; Quinlan, et al., 2011; Takahashi, et al., 2013; Vashi, et al., 2013). For example, a study by Takahashi et al. (2013) found that 30-day readmission for patients without care-transition interventions were 10.5 percent compared to no readmissions for those with a care intervention; emergency department admissions were 11.8 percent for the intervention group and 31.6 percent for those with no intervention.

Similar findings were reported by Dedhia and colleagues (2009), where 30-day post-discharge emergency department visits were 14 percent for patients with a transitions intervention and 21% for those without. Similarly, hospital readmissions were 14% with transition intervention and 22% without transition intervention. A clear consequence of no transitional care, which makes older adults vulnerable, is readmission to a new or previous care setting.

Potential Negative Health Outcomes

The second consequence of inadequate continuity of care and poor communication and coordination among providers and patients is the potential for negative health outcomes. Illness and injury that lead to hospitalization and the subsequent transitions from one care setting to another contribute to worsening decline among all levels of function, that is, no disability to severe disability (Gill et al., 2010). Consequences of transitions and potential for harm are particularly relevant to older adults who are taking multiple medications to treat chronic diseases (Foust et al., 2012; Gleason et al., 2010; Hu et al., 2012). Without proper transitional care, older adults are at risk for significant harm related to their medication regimes.

Gleason and colleagues found that "among 309 prescription medication order errors, 4 (1.3%) were rated as involving potentially longer hospitalization, 32 (10.4%) rated as potentially causing temporary harm, and 163 (52.4%) rated as potentially requiring increased monitoring or intervention to preclude harm" (p. 444). Potential medication harm during transitions can be particularly concerning for older adults with specific diseases that require close monitoring and management. Among heart failure patients discharged from the hospital, a study by Foust et al. (2012) found that a majority were discharged home with inconsistent or incomplete discharge instructions regarding their medications, and that a majority of the medications were high risk, previously associated with adverse events.

DEFINITION OF THE CONCEPT AND DISCUSSION

Vulnerability during transitions for older adults is defined as the inadequate continuity of care and poor communication and coordination among health care providers and patients and their families. Contributing to older adults' vulnerable state during transitions is taking multiple medications, as well as the fragmented nature of the United States health care system. Consequences of vulnerable transitions include readmissions to previous or new care settings and the potential for poor health outcomes.

Older adults are the highest consumers of health care services in the country and have many special and unique care needs. These realities, coupled with older adults' multiple care setting transitions and life event transitions, create opportunities for vulnerability. To achieve the best possible outcomes, we must ensure that all health care providers, and especially nurses, have the requisite KSAs to provide high-quality care (Esterson, Bazile, Mezey, Cortes, & Huba, 2013).

The NLN ACE.S project aims to facilitate nurses and faculty obtaining these unique older-adult-focused KSAs. Part of the knowledge necessary to provide high quality care to older adults is to understand what vulnerabilities older adults' face when making transitions.

The concept of vulnerability during transitions, which is part of the NLN ACE.S framework, provides a reference from which nursing faculty and students can begin to understand the experiences older adults face when transitioning from one setting to the next. Having awareness of how taking multiple medications and the fragmentation of the health care system contribute to inadequate continuity of care and poor communication and coordination among providers and patients is crucial. Further, the knowledge that vulnerabilities can lead to readmissions or negative health outcomes provides nurses with the knowledge and ability to take action and proactively prevent potential readmissions or negative outcomes. In clinical teaching settings where older adults are discharged home, nursing students with KSAs related to vulnerabilities during transitions may focus on ensuring patients have a clear understanding of discharge medication regimens and follow-up appointments with their primary-care providers.

This analysis was conducted on current health care literature found in two major bibliographic databases. However, what is evident from the analysis of the literature is that very few studies have focused on a broader interpretation of the concept of transitions. Most of the articles found in the body of literature related physical transitions between known care settings, such as hospital to home or hospital to nursing home, to emergency department and back to home. This provides valuable insights into the current focus and emphasis on care for older adults. It also provides insight into areas of health care that are significantly understudied and valued in the current healthcare climate, for example, the psychosocial aspects of aging and the impact of aging on well-being, versus medical disease outcome measures or financial impacts of health care utilization.

Further exploration and research are needed into how life transitions, such as losing a loved one, the inability to perform activities of daily living due to functional or cognitive decline, or transitioning into the role of grandparent or respected elder affect the risk for vulnerability in older adults. As the health care system evolves, additional work should be conducted to see how older adults' vulnerabilities change during transitions. Better and more effective means of communication through the use of smartphone technology may decrease vulnerabilities related to communication and coordination, whereas advances in gene therapy may create new and yet to be identified vulnerabilities in older adults.

CONCLUSION

This article defined the concept of vulnerability during transitions, which is part of the NLN ACE.S framework. Two antecedents were identified (use of multiple medications to treat disease, fragmentation of the health care system), two attributes (inadequate continuity of care, poor communication and coordination of care among health care providers and patients and their families), and two consequences (readmission to a previous or new care setting, potential negative health outcomes). An understanding of how this concept impacts older adults will facilitate high-quality care in a variety of health care settings. As the nursing profession embarks on the challenge of incorporating care of older adults as core nursing knowledge to be part of every curriculum, the NLN ACE.S framework and the concepts embedded within provide a useful and practical guide to facilitate this process.

*This scholarly project was funded by the Independence Foundation of Philadelphia.

References

American Association of Colleges of Nursing. (2008). *Essentials of Baccalaureate Education for Professional Nursing Practice*. Retrieved from http://www.aacn.nche.edu/education-resources/BaccEssentials08.pdf

American Association of Colleges of Nursing. (2010). *Recommended baccalaureate competencies and curricular guidelines for the nursing care of older adults: A supplement to the Essentials of Baccalaureate Education for Professional Nursing Practice*. Retrieved from www.aacn.nche.edu/geriatric-nursing/AACN_Gerocompetencies.pdf

Arora, V. M., Prochaska, M. L., Farnan, J. M., D'Arcy, M., Schwanz, K. J., Vinci, L. M., . . . & Johnson, J. K. (2010). Problems after discharge and understanding of communication with the PCPs among hospitalized seniors: A mixed methods study. *Journal of Hospital Medicine, 5*(7), 385–391. doi: 10.1002/jhm.668

Berman, A., Mezey, M., Kobayashi, M., Fulmer, T., Stanley, J., Thornlow, D., & Rosenfeld, P. (2005). Gerontological nursing content in baccalaureate nursing programs: Comparison of findings from 1997 and 2003. *Journal of Professional Nursing, 21*(5), 268–275. doi: 10.1016/j.profnurs.2005.07.005

Boltz, M., Parke, B., Shuluk, J., Capezuti, E., & Galvin, J. E. (2013). Care of the older adult in the emergency department: Nurses views of the pressing issues. *The Gerontologist, 53*(4), 441–453. doi:10.1093/geront/gnt004

Boxer, R. S., Dolansky, M. A., Frantz, M. A., Prosser, R., Hitch, J. A., & Pina, I. L. (2012). The bridge project improving heart failure care in skilled nursing facilities. *Journal of the American Medical Directors Association, 13*(1), 83.e1–83.e7. doi:10.1016/j.jamda.2011.01.005

Callahan, C. M., Arling, G., Tu, W., Rosenman, M. B., Counsell, S. R., Stump, T. E., & Hendrie, H. C. (2010). Transitions in care among older adults with and without dementia. *Journal of the American Geriatrics Society, 60*(5), 813–820. doi:10.1001/archinte.166.17.1822

Cline, D. D. (2014). A concept analysis of individualized aging. *Nursing Education Perspectives, 35*(3), 185–192. doi:10.5480/12–1053.1

Cline, D. D. (2015). Complexity of care: A concept analysis of older adult healthcare experiences. *Nursing Education Perspectives, 36*(2), 108–113. doi:10.5480/14–1362

Dedhia, P., Kravet, S., Bulger, J. L., Hinson, T., Sridharan, A., Kolodner, K., . . . & Howell, E. (2009). A quality improvement intervention to facilitate the transition of older adults from three hospitals back to their homes. *Journal of the American Geriatrics Society, 57*(9), 1540–1546. doi: 10.1111/j.1532–5415.2009.02430.x

Enguidanos, S., Gibbs, N., & Jamison, P. (2012). From hospital to home: A brief nurse practitioner intervention for vulnerable older adults. *Journal of Gerontological Nursing, 38*(3), 40–50. doi:10.3928/00989134–20120116–01

Esterson, J., Bazile, Y., Mezey, M., Cortes, T. A., & Huba, G. J. (2013). Ensuring specialty nurse competence to care for older adults. *Journal of Nursing Administration, 43*(10), 517–523. doi:10.1097/NNA.0b013e3182a3e870

Foust, J. B., Naylor, M. D., Bixby, B., & Ratcliffe, S. J. (2012). Medication problems occurring at hospital discharge among older adults with heart failure. *Research in Gerontological Nursing, 5*(1), 25–33. doi:10.3928/19404921–20111206–04

Gilje, F., Lacey, L., & Moore, C. (2007). Gerontology and geriatric issues and trends in U.S. nursing programs: A national survey. *Journal of Professional Nursing, 23*(1), 21–29. doi:10.1016/j.profnurs.2006.12.001

Gill, T. M., Allore, H. G., Gahbauer, E. A., & Murphy, T. E. (2010). Change in disability after hospitalization or restricted activity in older persons. *Journal of the American Medical Association, 304*(17), 1919–1928. doi: 10.1001/jama.2010.1568

Gleason, K. M., McDaniel, M. R., Feinglass, J., Baker, D. W., Lindquist, L., Liss, D., & Noskin, G. A. (2010). Results of the medications at transitions and clinical handoffs (MATCH) study: An analysis of medication reconciliation errors and risk factors at hospital admissions. *Journal of General Internal Medicine, 25*(5), 441–447. doi:10.1007/s11606-010-1256-6

Hu, S. H., Capezuti, E., Foust, J., B., Boltz, M. P., & Kim, H. (2012). Medication discrepancy and potentially inappropriate medication in older Chinese-American home-care patients after hospital discharge. *The American Journal of Geriatric Pharmacotherapy, 10*(5), 284–295. doi: 10.1016/j.amjopharm.2012.08.001

Institute of Medicine. (2008). *Retooling for an aging America: Building the health care workforce.* Washington, DC: National Academies Press.

Ironside, P. M., Tagliareni, M. E., McLaughlin, B., King, E., & Mengel, A. (2010). Fostering geriatrics in associate degree nursing education: An assessment of current curricula and clinical experiences. *Journal of Nursing Education, 49*(5), 246–252. doi: 10.3928/01484834-20100217-01

Latimer, D. G., & Thornlow, D. K. (2006). Incorporating geriatrics into baccalaureate nursing curricula: Laying the groundwork with faculty development. *Journal of Professional Nursing, 22*(2), 79–83. doi: 10.1016/j.profnurs.2006.01.012

Manski, R. J., Moeller, J. F., Chen, H., St. Clair, P. A., Schimmel, J., Magder, L. S., & Pepper, J. V. (2009). Dental coverage transitions. *American Journal of Managed Care, 15*(10), 729–735.

Manski, R. J., Moeller, J. F., St. Clair, P. A., Chen, H., Schimmel, J., & Pepper, J. V. (2011). The influence of changes in dental care coverage on dental care utilization among retirees and near-retirees in the United States, 2004–2006. *American Journal of Public Health, 101*(10), 1882–1891. doi:10.2105/AJPH.2011.300227

McNabney, M. K., Willging, P. R., Fried, L. P., & Durso, S. C. (2009). The "continuum of care" for older adults: Design and evaluation of an educational series. *Journal of the American Geriatrics Society, 57,* 1088–1095. doi: 10.1111/j.1532-5415.2009.02275.x

Nahm, E., Resnick, B., Orwig, D., Magaziner, J., & DeGrezia, M. (2010). Exploration of informal caregiving following hip fractures. *Geriatric Nursing, 31*(4), 1–13. doi: 10.1016/j.gerinurse.2010.01.003

Naylor, M. D., Kurtzman, E. T., Grabowski, D. C., Harrington, C., McClellan, M., & Reinhard, S. C. (2012). Unintended consequences of steps to cut readmissions and reform payment may threaten care of vulnerable older adults. *Health Affairs, 31*(7), 1623–1632. doi: 10.1377/hlthaff.2012.0110

Parrish, M. M., O'Malley, K., Adams, R. I., Adams, S. R., & Coleman, E. (2009). Implementation of the care transitions intervention: Sustainability and lessons learned. *Professional Case Management, 14*(6), 282–293. doi: 10.1097/NCM.0b013e3181c3d380

Parry, C., Min, S., Chugh, A., Chalmers, S., & Coleman, E. (2009). Further application of the care transitions intervention: Results of a randomized controlled trial conducted in a fee-for-service setting. *Home Health Care Services Quarterly, 28,* 84–99. doi: 10.1080/01621420903155924

Purdy, I. B. (2004). Vulnerable: A concept analysis. *Nursing Forum, 39*(4), 25–33.

Quinlan, N., Marcantonio, E. R., Inouye, S. K., Gill, T. M., Kamholz, B., & Rudolph, J. L. (2011). Vulnerability: The crossroads of frailty and delirium. *Journal of the American Geriatrics Society, 59*(Suppl 2), S262-S268. doi: 10.1111/j.1532-5415.2011.03674.x

Rogers, B. L., & Knafl, K. A. (2000). *Concept development in nursing: Foundations, techniques, and applications* (2nd ed.). Philadelphia, PA: Saunders.

Rose, A. J., Miller D. R., Ozonoff, A., Berlowitz, D. R., Ash, A. S., Zhao, S., . . . Hylek, E. M. (2013). Gaps in monitoring during oral anticoagulation. *Chest, 143*(3), 1–12. doi: 10.1378/chest.12-1119

Rose, K. M., & Lopez, R. P. (2012). Transitions in dementia care: Theoretical support for nursing roles. *Online Journal of Issues in Nursing, 17*(2), 1–19. doi: 10.3912/OJIN.Vol17No02Man04

Sharma, G., Freeman, J., Zhang, D., & Goodwin, J. S. (2009). Continuity of care and intensive care unit use at the end of life. *Archives of Internal Medicine, 169*(1), 81–86. doi: 10.1001/archinternmed.2008.514

Shippee, T. P. (2009). "But I am not moving": Residents' perspectives on transitions within a continuing care retirement community. *The Gerontologist, 49*(3), 418–426. doi: 10.1093/geront/gnp030

Tagliareni, M. E., Cline, D. D., Mengel, A., McLaughlin, B., & King, E. (2012). Quality care for older adults: The NLN Advancing Care Excellence for Seniors (ACE.S) Project. *Nursing Education Perspectives, 33*(3), 144–149. doi: 10.5480/1536–5026–33.3.144

Takahashi, P. Y., Haas, L. R., Quigg, S. M., Croghan, I. T., Naessens, J., M., Shah, N. D., & Hanson, G. J. (2013). 30-day hospital readmission of older adults using care transitions after hospitalization: A pilot prospective cohort study. *Clinical Interventions in Aging, 8*, 729–736. doi: 10.2147/CIA.S44390

Teno, J. M., Gozalo, P. L., Bynum, J. P., Leland, N. E., Miller, S. C., Morden, N. E., . . . & Mor, V. (2013). Change in end-of-life care for Medicare beneficiaries: Site of death, place of care, and health care transitions in 2000, 2005, and 2009. *Journal of the American Medical Association, 309*(5), 470–477. doi: 10.1001/jama.2012.207624

Terrell, K. M., Hustey, F. M., Hwang, U., Gerson, L. W., Wenger, N. S., & Miller, D. K. (2009). Quality indicators for geriatric emergency care. *Academic Emergency Medicine, 16*, 441–449. doi: 10.1111/j.1553–2712.2009.00382.x

Toles, M., Barroso, J., Colon-Emeric, C., Corazzini, K., McConnell, E., & Anderson, R. A. (2012). Staff interaction strategies that optimize delivery of transitional care in a skilled nursing facility: A multiple case study. *Family & Community Health, 35*(4), 334–344. doi: 10.1097/FCH.0b013e31826666eb

Tomm-Bonde, L. (2012). The naïve nurse: Revisiting vulnerability for nursing. *BMC Nursing, 11*(5), 1–7. doi:10.1186/1472–6955–11–5

Vashi, A. A., Fox, J. P., Carr, B. G., D'Onofrio, G., Pines, M. J., Ross, J. S., & Gross, C. P. (2013). Use of hospital-based acute care among patients recently discharged from the hospital. *Journal of the American Medical Association, 309*(4), 364–371.

5

Gerontological Nursing Content in General Medical/Surgical Textbooks: Where Is It?

Daniel D. Cline, PhD, RN
Jeannette Manchester, DNP, RN
M. Elaine Tagliareni, EdD, RN, CNE, FAAN

ABSTRACT

To provide quality care to the rapidly growing aging population, nursing education will need to be transformed. Although several approaches will be used to meet this challenge, fundamental to most nursing programs is the use of a general medical/surgical nursing textbook. This article examines the quantity and quality of gerontological nursing content found in five general medical/surgical nursing textbooks published between 2009 and 2011. The analysis shows that gerontological nursing content is poorly covered and of low quality. The findings point to the need to work with publishers to improve the quality and depth of content related to care of older adults in nursing textbooks.

Since the original publication of this paper (Cline, Manchester, & Tagliareni, 2012), three of the medical/surgical textbooks printed new editions. New publications came out in 2014 and 2016. These three recent publications were reviewed and compared to the original analysis to see if there had been significant changes. Unfortunately, few differences were identified in the new editions from the previous editions—leading to continued concern with the quality and quantity of gerontological content in nursing medical/surgical textbooks.

Rapid growth in the population of adults aged 65 years or older in the United States (Administration on Aging, 2009) has significant implications for the education of health care providers (Institute of Medicine [IOM], 2003). Older adults are the largest consumers of health care services and, in 2007, accounted for 24 percent of all inpatient admissions (DeFrances, Lucas, Buie, & Golosinskiy, 2008). To meet the needs of this population, the IOM recommends that systems of care be redesigned to optimize quality (2001, 2004). Further, the IOM emphasizes the need to address the shortage of qualified health care providers (2008) and focus on the unique needs of older adults (2003).

Currently, all health professions (e.g., registered nurses, physicians, dentists, pharmacists) face the challenge of educating graduates with expertise in the care of older adults (IOM, 2008). In nursing education, leading organizations have made gerontological education a priority, as evidenced by the National League for Nursing's (NLN) vision statement, *Caring for Older Adults* (2012), and the American Association of Colleges of Nursing's (AACN) *Recommended Baccalaureate Competencies and Curricular Guidelines for the Nursing Care of Older Adults* (2010).

A challenge facing nursing education has been the failure of pre-licensure programs to focus curricula on the unique and complex needs of older adults. Less obvious, but no less important, is the lack of appropriate content on care of older adults in contemporary health sciences textbooks.

As pedagogies are developed for health professionals of all types to gain expertise in the care of older adults, textbooks will likely be foundational for many learning experiences. General medical/surgical nursing textbooks are widely used in pre-licensure nursing programs as a principal reference source for students' acquisition of knowledge regarding disease pathophysiology, treatment regimens, and appropriate nursing care of hospitalized patients. The purpose of this analysis was to examine the amount and quality of gerontological nursing content in a sample of currently available general medical/surgical nursing (GMSN) textbooks published by four large and well-established health science publishing companies.

REVIEW OF THE LITERATURE
Gerontological Content in Nursing Curricula

Nurses are the largest group of health care providers in the United States and spend more time with patients in more settings than any other discipline. Thus, inadequate gerontological content in nursing education (Gilje, Lacey, & Moore, 2007; IOM, 2008; Ironside, Tagliareni, McLaughlin, King, & Mengel, 2010) is of particular concern.

Although most registered nurses (RNs) provide care to older adults, only a third of all baccalaureate nursing schools (BSN) accredited by the AACN in 2003 offered a stand-alone gerontology course (Berman et al., 2005). Further, in 2004, 25 percent of BSN schools did not have an expert gerontological nurse faculty member (Berman et al., 2005). A recent national survey of associate degree nursing (ADN) programs showed that content related to care of older adults comprised only 10 percent to 25 percent of curricular content (Ironside et al., 2010). According to the most recent workforce data, approximately 45 percent of RNs are educated in associate degree programs (U.S. Department of Health and Human Services, 2010), indicating a significant gap in the geriatric education of the RN workforce.

A key difficulty related to increasing geriatric content in schools of nursing is a shortage of faculty prepared in gerontology (Gilje et al., 2007). The vast majority of respondents to a 2004 survey indicated that their school had no faculty certified through the American Nurse Credentialing Center (ANCC) as a gerontological RN (91.5 percent), nurse practitioner (76 percent), or clinical nurse specialist (85 percent). Of 110 public institutions offering nursing degrees, only 76 individual faculty members were identified as ANCC-certified in geriatrics as an RN, nurse practitioner, or clinical nurse specialist. In the 92 private institutions offering a baccalaureate nursing degree, only 31 individual faculty members were identified as certified in these same areas (Gilje et al., 2007).

A study by Gilje et al. (2007) showed that about half (51 percent) of baccalaureate-degree-granting schools of nursing offered a course in geriatrics; 49 percent indicated they offered geriatric content through an integrated format. Gilje et al.'s finding is an improvement over Berman et al.'s finding (2005) that only a third of programs offered a stand-alone course. Of the programs reported by Gilje et al. to offer a stand-alone geriatric course, only 44 included a clinical component with the course.

A study by Ironside et al. (2010) found that in ADN programs, only 5 percent of schools surveyed offered stand-alone geriatric specialty courses or experiences. Also the study's finding that nearly 60 percent of respondents "were unfamiliar with newer geriatric resources" (p. 250) was of particular concern. Respondents were unfamiliar with resources available from the John A. Hartford Foundation, the *American Journal of Nursing* series known as "A New Look at the Old," and the AACN baccalaureate competencies and curricular guidelines for geriatric nursing (Ironside et al.). Without faculty experts to lead the curricular change, it will be difficult to increase the basic geriatric knowledge of all nurses.

Specialty Content in Nursing Textbooks

Several articles published since 2000 examined and reviewed specialty content in nursing textbooks related to the care of older adults. Topics included: pressure ulcers (Ayello & Meaney, 2003); end-of-life (EOL) care (Kirchhoff, Beckstrand, & Anumandla, 2003); pain management during EOL care (Ferrell, Virani, Grant, Vallerand, & McCaffery, 2000); spirituality and spiritual care (McEwen, 2004; Pesut, 2008); and disability-related content (Smeltzer, Robinson-Smith, Dolen, Duffin, & Al-Maqbali, 2010). These reviews were conducted for a variety of reasons: to increase knowledge and development in advancing fields of science; to identify needs within the nursing profession for greater awareness in certain areas; and to replicate previous studies, to determine if textbooks are incorporating the latest evidence in emerging care and treatment options.

Changes in best practices occur frequently as new therapies are discovered that lead to improved outcomes. Ayello and Meaney (2003) sought to replicate a 1993 study to determine if nursing textbooks were up to date with the rapid increase in knowledge and changes in the care of pressure ulcers that happened between 1993 and 2003. They found wide variation in the eight textbooks reviewed; however, they did find increased emphasis on current treatment and discussion of research-based nursing care of pressure ulcers in all textbooks. They recommended that a full chapter be dedicated to pressure ulcer care in all texts to adequately cover the topic.

Reviews by Kirchoff et al. (2003) and Ferrell et al. (2000) focused on EOL content. Kirchoff and Beckstrand focused specifically on pain management at the end of life. They examined 14 critical-care nursing textbooks for eight content areas identified as undergraduate competencies by the AACN and four additional topic areas considered integral to EOL care. As none of the texts they reviewed had content in all 12 specified areas, the authors concluded there is significant need for improved EOL content in critical care nursing textbooks. Similarly, in their review of pain management at the end of life, Ferrell et al. found "significant deficits in nursing texts, both in the absence of essential information and in the presence of inaccurate information" (p. 226).

Two reviews focused on spirituality and spiritual care. The first review, by McEwen (2004), sought to analyze nursing textbooks (medical/surgical, fundamentals, psychiatric, maternal/child, and others) to determine where spirituality is discussed and its adequacy. Most relevant to this review, McEwen found that "very minimal attention was given to spiritual care in medical/surgical nursing books" (p. 25), and in gerontological nursing textbooks, it varied; however, content in the nursing fundamentals texts was comprehensive. Building on McEwen's work (2004), Pesut (2008) focused specifically on nursing fundamentals textbooks. These were found to have a comprehensive review of the content, but issues regarding spirituality were presented as conceptual and often led to dichotomies for students, for example, religion versus spirituality.

Smeltzer et al. (2010) reviewed disability-related content in nursing textbooks. They concluded that the absence of such content was significant given the aging population and the growing number of people with disabilities. They recommended that until the content in nursing textbooks improves, nurse educators must use additional resources to teach disability-related content.

No reviews were found looking specifically at gerontological nursing content. Given the lack of geriatric-prepared faculty and geriatric specialty courses in pre-licensure nursing programs, GMSN textbooks may be a significant resource for pre-licensure nursing students regarding knowledge related to gerontological nursing. Therefore, a review of GMSN textbooks is warranted and needed.

An important theme found in each of the reviews cited was that nursing textbooks often lack sufficient content or have poor coverage of a variety of specialty topics. This analysis of GMSN textbooks will help determine if this theme is true for gerontological content as well.

METHOD

This review of gerontological nursing content in GMSN textbooks resulted from work related to the NLN's Advancing Care Excellence for Seniors (ACE.S) project. The framework for analysis of the GSMN textbooks was structured around nursing protocols for best practices identified in *Evidence-Based Geriatric Nursing Protocols for Best Practice* (Capezuti et al., 2008), a leading reference on geriatric acute care nursing edited by recognized leaders in the field of gerontological nursing. Capezuti et al. provide guidelines on specific geriatric nursing topics developed by experts and based on current best evidence. Each chapter, or topical area from the text, was developed using the Instrument for Appraisal of Guidelines for Research & Evaluation (AGREE) (www.agreetrust.org) to rate the level of evidence for the topic, thereby creating a rigorous and systematic literature review process and ensuring protocols for best practice included in the text were based on the best available evidence.

The next step in the analysis involved an extensive review of five GMSN textbooks published between 2009 and 2012 and currently available for use in pre-licensure nursing programs. (See Table 5.1.) The textbooks were published by four large health sciences publishing companies. The first author reviewed each textbook for content related to the previously identified topic areas. Topic content was identified and located in the textbook by: (a) searching the index for key words, (b) reviewing chapters with relevant content, and (c) reading chapters identified as specific to medical/surgical care of

TABLE 5.1	
Medical/Surgical and Gerontology Textbooks Used in the Review	
Medical/Surgical Nursing	**Author(s)/Year of Publication**
Medical-Surgical Nursing: Clinical Management for Positive Outcomes	J. M. Black & J. H. Hawks (2009)
Contemporary Medical-Surgical Nursing (2nd ed.)	R. Daniels & L. Nicoll (2012)
Medical-Surgical Nursing: Patient Centered Collaborative Care	D. D. Ignatvicius & M. L. Workman (2010) (2016)
Medical Surgical Nursing: Assessment and Management of Clinical Problems	S. L. Lewis, S. R. Dirksen, M. M. Heitkemper, L. Bucher, & I. M. Camera (2011) (2014)
Brunner and Suddarth's Textbook of Medical-Surgical Nursing	S. C. Smeltzer, J. L. Hinkle, B. Bare, & K. H. Cheever (2010) J. L. Hinkle, K. H. Cheever (2014)
Gerontological Specific	**Authors**
Evidence-Based Geriatric Nursing Protocols for Best Practice	E. C. Capezuti, D. Zwicker, M. Mezey, T. Fulmer, D. Gray-Miceli, & M. Kluger (2008)
Gerontological Nursing	C. Eliopoulos (2010)
Gerontological Nursing: The Essential Guide to Clinical Practice	P. A. Tabloski (2010)
Ebersole and Hess' Gerontological Nursing & Healthy Aging	T. A. Touhy & K. F. Jet (2010)

older adults. This review process was repeated by the second author. The two authors then discussed areas where there were discrepancies and came to agreement on rating the amount and quality of the content.

To strengthen the analysis and provide rigor, topical areas relevant to the care of older adults not identified by Capezuti et al. (2008), but identified in the GMSN textbooks, were included in the analysis matrix as topic areas. Two additional areas were identified: palliative care and infection. This resulted in total of 29 topic areas. (See Table 5.2.)

Each of the 29 topical areas was then cross-referenced with three textbooks specializing in gerontological nursing, all published in 2010 by three of the same large publishing companies. This was done to ensure that the 29 topical areas identified were significant throughout the literature and to provide cross-reference regarding the amount and quality of content found in the general medical/surgical nursing textbooks.

FINDINGS

The review of five current general medical/surgical nursing textbooks and four gerontology-specific nursing textbooks revealed a concerning trend. The publishing companies represented in this review had access to appropriate and high-quality gerontological nursing content, as evident in the gerontological textbooks, but did not include

TABLE 5.2

Evaluation of Gerontological Content in Five General Medical/ Surgical Nursing Textbooks by Topic Area

Topic Area	Superior/Good	Adequate/Fair	Inadequate/Poor
Assessment of Function	0	1	4
Assessment of Cognitive Function	0	1	4
Depression	0	2	3
Dementia	4	1	0
Delirium	1	2	2
Family Care giving	0	1	4
Preventing Falls	0	0	5
Pain Management	1	3	1
Iatrogenisis	0	0	5
Reducing Adverse Drug Events/ (Polypharmacy)	0	1	4
Urinary Incontinence	0	1	4
Mealtime Difficulties	0	0	5
Nutrition	0	0	5
Managing Oral Hydration	0	0	5
Oral Health Care	0	0	5
Preventing Pressure Ulcers and Skin Tears	0	5	0
Sleep	0	1	4
Sensory Changes	1	1	3
Physical Restraints and Side Rails	0	0	5
Health Care Decision Making	0	3	2
Advanced Directives	0	3	2
Assessment and Management of the Critically Ill	0	0	5
Fluid Overload: Managing HF Patients	0	0	5
Cancer Assessment and Intervention Strategies	0	0	5
Issues Regarding Sexuality	0	0	5
Substance Misuse and Alcohol Use Disorders	0	0	5
Palliative Care	5	1	1
Infection	0	1	4

Note: This table lists 29 topic areas of gerontological nursing content evaluated in five general medical/surgical nursing textbooks and ranked as Superior/Good, Adequate/Fair, or Inadequate/Poor.

such content in their general medical/surgical texts. Specifically, the gerontological content in the medical/surgical texts was poorly covered, while the content in the specialty texts provided an excellent review of pertinent care of older adults. GMSN textbooks, perhaps the most widely used knowledge-dissemination tool for the care of hospitalized older adults in pre-licensure nursing programs, appeared to present gerontological content as disease progression or health problems, an approach that may convey a negative impression of aging and older adults for pre-licensure nursing students.

The GMSN textbooks were specifically examined for amount and quality of gerontological nursing content based on 29 topic areas relevant to quality care for hospitalized older adults. Content was ranked as either: (a) inadequate coverage and poor quality; (b) adequate coverage and fair quality; or (c) superior coverage and good quality. (See Table 5.2.)

"Inadequate coverage and poor quality" indicated that the topic area was either completely absent, briefly covered, or lacked a specific focus on older adults. For example, one GMSN text that dedicated a full chapter on health problems of older adults had no content on sexuality.

"Adequate coverage and fair quality" indicated that the topic was appropriately covered, but lacked depth and breadth, thereby providing readers with cursory knowledge of the subject. For example, some GMSN texts, at the end of several pages related to a specific disease process, have a short (two- to three-paragraph) section focused on gerontological considerations. While important knowledge is conveyed to the reader, the amount of information is limited and the quality of the content is superficial. The three additional GMSN textbooks published in 2014 and 2016 continued the trend seen in previous editions with gerontological content at the end of the section or in a table/chart. Cursory knowledge is problematic as novice nurses may equate lack of depth or breadth on a topic with lacking clinical importance. Further, including gerontological content at the end of a section in a cursory way may lead students to perceive it as having little value.

"Superior content and good quality" indicated the topic was covered in depth and provided a solid foundation from which to base future nursing actions. For example, all GMSN textbooks had an entire chapter dedicated to palliative care that covered the topic in depth, with information on patient and family issues, symptom management, and other psychosocial issues surrounding palliative care. While palliative care is not needed only by older adults, older adults frequently use palliative care services and have special palliative care needs (Kapo, Morrison, & Liao, 2007).

The rankings for the 29 topics are included in Table 5.2. Twelve topic areas had inadequate content and poor quality in each of the five textbooks. These included important topics such as prevention of falls, nutrition, oral health, issues regarding sexuality, and substance and alcohol use disorders. Eight topics were labeled inadequate content and poor quality areas in four of the five GMSN textbooks. Two topics, sensory changes and depression, were labeled inadequate content and poor quality in three of the five textbooks. Twenty-two of the 29 topics, or 75 percent of the GMSN textbooks had inadequate content and poor quality in three of the five textbooks reviewed.

Only six topic areas were labeled adequate coverage and fair quality in three of the five textbooks: delirium, pain management, pressure ulcers/skin, health care decision-making, advanced directives, and palliative care. Interestingly, all of the textbooks had adequate coverage and fair quality with regard to preventing pressure ulcers/skin tears and superior content and good quality with regard to palliative care. Among the GMSN textbooks, only one topic area was labeled superior content and good quality, in contrast to nearly all of the 29 topic areas in the four subject-specific nursing textbooks.

DISCUSSION

Improving the care of older adults will require transforming our health care system in several ways, including improving access to care, changing the settings in which care is delivered, shifting the focus from acute to chronic care, improving quality and safety, and changing how health care providers are educated. Too few nursing faculty have expertise in gerontological nursing. The number of faculty with gerontological expertise and the amount of gerontological nursing content provided in pre-licensure programs must be increased to ensure that graduates have the necessary knowledge, skills, and attitudes to provide high-quality care to older adults.

According to Kovner, Mezey, and Harrington (2002), there is approximately one geriatric-educated provider for every 2000 people over the age of 65 years old in the United States. However, Kovner and colleagues do not believe that geriatric specialists, such as geriatricians or geriatric nurse practitioners, are the only providers who can provide quality care to the aging population. One approach they suggest is for the entire health care workforce to receive basic education in geriatrics, just as students receive education in pediatrics. If that were to happen, a need would still exist to increase the number of geriatric specialists for consultations, but the use of technology (e.g., email or telemedicine) would allow many providers, and the patients they care for, access to a geriatric specialist.

Broad-based gerontological education as an approach to increase the number of nurse providers with the requisite gerontological knowledge has been put into policy through the National Council State Boards of Nursing Consensus Model. The new advanced practice nursing model eliminates the geriatric nurse practitioner and adult nurse practitioner subspecialty tracks and requires *all* nurse practitioner tracks to include content related to the care of older adults (AACN, 2012). Broad-based education in geriatrics has also been discussed for the education of physicians (Boult, Counsell, Leipzig, & Berenson, 2010).

Significant investments aimed at strengthening content related to care of older adults in nursing education have been made over the past 10 years. The John A. Hartford Foundation has led the way by funding initiatives such as the Hartford Institute for Geriatric Nursing at New York University, nine Hartford Geriatric Nurse Education Centers, and the Building Academic Geriatric Nursing Capacity (BAGNC) Scholar and Fellow Program. The impact of these programs on advancing gerontological nursing has been impressive. For example, BAGNC awardees have published 1,133 articles related to care of older adults, received more than 72 million dollars in federal and private foundation grant monies, and taught at least 11,052 undergraduate nursing students in courses where at least 50 percent of the course content was specific to gerontological nursing (Franklin et al., 2011).

Despite these impressive results, the majority of pre-licensure nursing programs continue to lack faculty with skills and expertise in gerontological nursing. Thus, the gerontological nursing content most students receive comes, in part, from the general medical/surgical nursing textbooks used to guide their studies.

In addition to the other initiatives, the John A. Hartford Foundation collaborated with the AACN and the Hartford Institute for Geriatric Nursing at New York University to develop *Recommended Baccalaureate Competencies and Curricular Guidelines for the Nursing Care of Older Adults* (AACN, 2010). This document contains 19 gerontological nursing competency statements and guidelines to "help nurse educators incorporate geriatric-focused nursing content and learning opportunities into the baccalaureate nursing curriculum, including both the didactic and clinical experiences" (p. 9). While competency statements and curricular guides are needed, they are not sufficient to change pre-licensure nursing education.

In an effort to increase the breadth of gerontological nursing content taught to pre-licensure nursing students, the John A. Hartford Foundation, the Independence Foundation, and the Laerdal Corporation funded a partnership between the NLN and Community College of Philadelphia that resulted in the NLN ACE.S project (www.nln.org/facultyprograms/facultyresources/aces/index.htm). This project aims to advance the care of older adults through improvement in gerontological nursing education. A variety of tools to facilitate faculty growth in gerontological nursing, including use of simulation, unfolding cases, and teaching strategies were developed and will be disseminated to 20 states through funding from the Hearst Foundations. However, like other initiatives, the NLN ACE.S project does not address the deficiencies in general medical/surgical nursing textbooks. Faculty who are well versed in gerontological nursing may design innovative teaching and learning strategies, and may create unique encounters for students with older adults, but at the end of the day, many students will open their general medical/surgical nursing textbook to prepare for their clinical experiences.

LIMITATIONS

There are limitations to this review. First, the original analysis only included five general medical/surgical nursing textbooks published from 2009–2012 and four gerontological nursing-specific textbooks. In 2016, three updated editions (published from 2014–2016) of the GMSN textbooks were also reviewed. Review of different textbooks could provide different findings. However, the five published general medical/surgical textbooks selected for review are from four of the largest publishers of health care textbooks and surely are typical of published textbooks in terms of the amount and quality of gerontological nursing content. This supposition is reinforced by the finding that there is little variation among the five texts. The framework used for the analysis was based on best practice in acute care, thereby excluding potentially important topic areas for the care of older adults in other settings such as assisted living, long-term care, and the community.

Another limitation inherent in any analysis of published textbooks is the amount of time it takes to get the book published. Textbooks will not have the most up-to-date evidence. However, since most curricula are not taught with the exclusive use of publications, which are more current than textbooks, it is appropriate to examine the content and quality of textbooks. As new editions are published they should be examined to determine the quality and quantity of gerontological nursing content.

CONCLUSIONS

To ensure optimal outcomes and good quality of life for the rapidly growing older adult population, significant changes to our current health care system and the education of health professional, including nurses, are needed. Important progress has been made related to increasing the number of nurse faculty with gerontological knowledge and expertise in pre-licensure and graduate nursing programs through the AACN's recommended competencies and guidelines and the BAGNC Scholars and Fellows program. However, it is profoundly concerning that the primary textbooks used as references and knowledge repositories for the care of hospitalized older adults, the general medical/surgical nursing textbooks, are severely deficient in both the amount and quality of gerontological nursing content.

The deficiencies found in this study should lead all nurse educators, researchers, and leaders to ask: "How is this so? How can we change this?" These are not easy questions to answer. However, the profession must work with publishing companies to ensure that nursing textbooks contain the information and knowledge new nurses need to deliver high quality care to our rapidly changing and aging population. Current textbooks are long and cumbersome. Given the move to electronic texts and the advent of new technologies, such as tablet computers, there may be options to increase the amount and quality of gerontological nursing content in medical/surgical nursing textbooks without adding to size or limiting portability. The use of technology may also make texts more interactive, thereby making their use more efficient and effective.

A final consideration is related to how curricular changes are integrated in schools of nursing. Without doubt, over the past 10 years, there has been significant progress made in providing gerontological nursing education to pre-licensure nursing students. The emphasis awareness of older adults' care needs has led to many schools of nursing to add a gerontological nursing course to pre-licensure curricula. However, schools of nursing need to be cautious to ensure gerontological nursing courses are not silo courses without meaningful integration into the medical/surgical core courses. The lack of gerontological nursing content and the presentation of that content in GMSN textbooks remains an area of concern and opportunity.

References

Administration on Aging. (2009). *A profile of older Americans: 2009.* U.S. Department of Health and Human Services. Retrieved from http://www.aoa.acl.gov/Aging_Statistics/Profile/2009/index.aspx

American Association of Colleges of Nursing. (2010). Recommended Baccalaureate Competencies and Curricular Guidelines for Geriatric Nursing Care. Retrieved from www.aacn.nche.edu/geriatric-nursing/AACN_Gerocompetencies.pdf

American Association of Colleges of Nursing. (2012). *APRN consensus process.* Retrieved from www.aacn.nche.edu/education-resources/aprn-consensus-process

Ayello, E., & Meaney, G. (2003). Replicating a survey of pressure ulcer content in nursing textbooks. *Journal of Wound, Ostomy, and Continence Nursing, 30*(5), 266–271. doi:10.1067/mjw.2003.147

Berman, A., Mezey, M., Kobayashi, M., Fulmer, T., Stanley, J., & Thornlow, D. (2005). Gerontological nursing content in baccalaureate nursing programs: Comparison of findings from 1997 and 2003. *Journal of Professional Nursing, 21*(5), 268–275. doi:10.1016/j. profnurs.2005.07.005

Boult, C., Counsell, S. R., Leipzig, R. M., & Berenson, R. A. (2010). The urgency of preparing primary care physicians to care for older people with chronic illness. *Health Affairs, 29*(5), 811–818. doi: 10.1377/hlthaff.2010.0095

Capezuti, E. C., Zwicker, D., Mezey, M., Fulmer, T. T., Gray-Miceli, D., & Kluger, M. (2008). *Evidence-based geriatric nursing protocols for best practice.* New York: Springer Publishing.

Cline, D., Manchester, J., Tagliareni, M.E. (2012). Gerontological Nursing Content in General Medical/Surgical Textbooks: Where Is It? *Nursing Education Perspectives, 33*(3), 150–155.

DeFrances, C. J., Lucas, C. A., Buie, V. C., & Golosinskiy, A. (2008, July 30). 2006 National Hospital Discharge Survey. *National Health Statistics Reports* (Number 5). Retrieved from www.cdc.gov/nchs/data/nhsr005.pdf

Ferrell, B., Virani, R., Grant, M., Vallerand, A., & McCaffery, M. (2000). Analysis of pain content in nursing textbooks. *Journal of Pain and Symptom Management, 19*(3), 216–228.

Franklin, P. D., Archbold, P. G., Fagin, C. M., Gail, E., Siegel, E., Sofaer, S., & Firminger, K. (2011). Building academic geriatric nursing capacity: Results after the first 10 years and implications for the future. *Nursing Outlook, 59*(4), 198–205. doi:10.1016/j. outlook.2011.05.011

Gilje, F., Lacey, L., & Moore, C. (2007). Gerontology and geriatric issues and trends in U.S. nursing programs: A national survey. *Journal of Professional Nursing, 23*(1), 21–29. doi:10.1016/j.profnurs.2006.12.001

Institute of Medicine. (2001). *Crossing the quality chasm: A new health system for the 21st century.* Washington, DC: National Academies Press.

Institute of Medicine. (2003). *Health professions education: A bridge to quality.* Washington, DC: National Academies Press.

Institute of Medicine. (2004). *Keeping patients safe: Transforming the work environment for nurses and patient safety.* Washington, DC: National Academies Press.

Institute of Medicine. (2008). *Retooling for an aging America: Building the health care work force.* Washington, DC: National Academies Press.

Ironside, P. M., Tagliareni, M. E., McLaughlin, B., King, E., & Mengel, A. (2010). Fostering geriatrics in associate degree nursing education: An assessment of current curricula and clinical experiences. *Journal of Nursing Education, 49*(5), 246–252. doi:10.3928/01484834–20100217–01

Kapo, J., Morrison, L. J., & Liao, S. (2007). Palliative care for the older adult. *Journal of Palliative Medicine, 10*(1), 185–209. doi: 10.1089/jpm.20069989

Kirchoff, K. T., Beckstrand, R. L., & Anumandla, P. R. (2003). Analysis of end-of-life content in critical care nursing textbooks. *Journal of Professional Nursing, 19*(6), 372–381. doi:10.1016/ S8755–7223(03)00141–8

Kovner, C., Mezey, M., & Harrington, C. (2002). Who cares for older adults? Workforce implications of an aging society. *Health Affairs, 21*(5), 78–89.

McEwen, M. (2004). Analysis of spirituality content in nursing textbooks. *Journal of Nursing Education, 43*(1), 20–30.

The National League for Nursing. (2012). Caring for older adults [NLN Vision Series]. Retrieved from http://www.nln.org/aboutnln/ livingdocuments/pdf/nlnvision_2.pdf

Pesut, B. (2008). Spirituality and spiritual care in nursing fundamentals textbooks. *Journal of Nursing Education, 47*(4), 167–173.

Smeltzer, S. C., Robinson-Smith, G., Dolen M. A., Duffin, J. M., & Al-Maqbali, M. (2010). Disability related content in nursing textbooks. *Nursing Education Perspectives, 31*(3), 148–155.

U.S. Department of Health and Human Services, Health Resources and Services Administration. (2010). *The registered nurse population: Findings from the 2008 National Sample Survey of Registered Nurses.* Retrieved from http://bhpr.hrsa.gov/ healthworkforce/rnsurveys/rnsurveyfinal.pdf

6

Integrating QSEN and ACE.S: An NLN Simulation Leader Project

Susan G. Forneris, PhD, RN, CNE, CHSE-A

JoAnn G. Crownover, DNP, RN, CNE

Laurie Dorsey, MSN, RN

Nancy B. Leahy, RN, MSN, CHSE

Nancy A. Maas, MSN, FNP-BC, CNE

Lorrie Wong, PhD, RN, CHSE-A

Anne Zabriskie, MS, RN, CNE

Jean Ellen Zavertnik, DNP, RN, ACNS-BC, CNE

ABSTRACT

Caring for the special needs of the aging adult is an increasingly important focus in nursing education. Knowledge continues to evolve, creating exciting learning opportunities for nursing students and challenges for nurse educators. One such challenge is to use simulation to operationalize knowledge around safe care of the aging adult.

The 2010–2011 National League for Nursing (NLN) Simulation Leader Curriculum Integration Team—nurse educators selected to participate in a year-long simulation leadership development program—examined key issues in the design, development, use, and integration of simulation in nursing education and incorporated their collaborative work on SIRC, the NLN Simulation Innovation Resource Center. The group noted that resources to guide faculty on how to tailor simulation to incorporate competencies around quality and safety in care of the aging are not easily accessible. This article provides an overview of the resources developed by the team. It is intended as a guide to incorporate concepts of quality and safety education for nurses into an unfolding simulation focused on care of the aging adult.

BACKGROUND

Quality and Safety Education for Nurses (QSEN) addresses the nursing competencies needed to assure the quality and safety of patient care. Adapted from the Institute of Medicine (IOM) competencies for nursing (2003), QSEN outlines essential features of competent nursing practice (nursing competencies) to improve patient safety and quality in health care settings. The six QSEN competencies are: Patient-Centered Care, Teamwork and Collaboration, Evidence-Based Practice, Quality Improvement, Safety, and Informatics (Cronenwett et al., 2007). Subsets of each QSEN competency include knowledge, skills, and attitudes achievable during the educational process. Results of the QSEN National Delphi Study (Barton, Armstrong, Preheim, Gelmon, & Andrus, 2009) led to the leveling of QSEN competencies into beginner, intermediate, and advanced learning objectives for integration across a nursing curriculum.

The use of an unfolding case study correlates well with a leveled approach in the teaching of quality and safety for care of the older adult. Unfolding case studies expose students to multiple aspects of a clinical situation and promote problem solving using an experiential learning method (Page, Kowlowitz, & Alden, 2010). The curriculum integration team determined that a scenario that unfolded over time would be an ideal simulation exemplar to demonstrate the integration of beginner-, intermediate-, and advance-level QSEN competencies in care of the aging adult client.

The NLN, in partnership with the Community College of Philadelphia and with funding from the John A. Hartford foundation, Laerdal Medical, and the Independence Foundation, developed the ACE.S (Advancing Care Excellence for Seniors) project to teach nursing students how to care for the older adults. The ACE.S project features four cases that unfold over time, take place in a variety of health care settings, and require complex decision-making. The team determined that blending QSEN with ACE.S was a natural choice for the focus of the project.

Millie Larsen (Reese, 2010), one of four ACE.S cases, includes a web-based text document with links to audio files and other supportive information. ACE.S provides teaching tools, evidence-based resources, and, importantly, a framework for incorporating the complexities of caring for the aging adult. Permission was granted by the NLN to utilize the ACE.S scenario featuring Millie for inclusion in the curriculum integration project.

Millie Larsen's case unfolds in three scenarios, with settings in an outpatient clinic and in an acute-care hospital. It concludes with conflict regarding discharge from the

TABLE 6.1

Integration of QSEN Competencies Leveled with ACE.S Millie Larsen Simulations

ACE.S Millie Larsen Unfolding Simulations	Overview of Unfolding Simulation	QSEN Competency Level
Simulation 1	3:00 PM—Initial admission to the hospital from the outpatient clinic.	Beginner QSEN competencies—FOCUS on Patient-Centered Care
Simulation 2	7:00 AM—Hospital stay Day 2	Intermediate QSEN competencies—FOCUS on Safety, Patient-Centered Care, Teamwork and Collaboration
Simulation 3	9:00 AM—Hospital stay Day 2: discharge planning	Advanced QSEN competencies—FOCUS on Safety, Patient-Centered Care, Teamwork and Collaboration, Quality Assurance, Informatics

inpatient setting. The scenarios reveal a compelling story illustrating the interaction of the multiple factors that affect a geriatric client's health. Table 6.1 illustrates how the simulation leader project integrated the QSEN competencies by level into Millie's unfolding health care encounters. The beginner competencies are integrated into Millie's initial admission simulation; the intermediate and advanced competencies are integrated into Millie's hospital stay and discharge simulations, respectively.

BEGINNER QSEN COMPETENCIES

The task of incorporating QSEN competencies into an existing curricular framework is daunting. However, it is possible to take an existing learning activity, identify the appropriate knowledge, skills, and attitudes (KSAs), and easily adapt it to the QSEN model.

Using the Millie Larsen unfolding case scenario, the Simulation Leadership Team examined each part of the case to identify existing or potential beginning-level competencies. Scenario 1 was examined without changes to the original ACE.S Simulation Design Template, demonstrating how an existing simulation can be utilized without modification. Scenarios 2 and 3 were adapted, with simple variations, to incorporate more competencies or concentrate on a specific domain. Furthermore, the scenarios were delineated for progression from simple to complex KSAs, as developed by the national Delphi study (Barton et al., 2009).

The QSEN competency focused on Patient-Centered Care is a foundational concept essential for beginning nursing students. Millie's introductory monologue and Scenario 1 are easily utilized for an introductory nursing course, and the competencies are identified without difficulty. Table 6.2 illustrates beginner-level Patient-Centered Care KSAs for demonstration in Millie's outpatient simulation (Scenario 1).

INTERMEDIATE QSEN COMPETENCIES

Millie Larsen's situation unfolds further in simulation scenario 2 with her admission to an acute-care facility. This scenario was adapted to introduce several intermediate QSEN level concerns that the student must address (e.g., Millie's fall; a medication near-miss surrounding an unclear change in medication dosing; an outside phone call inquiry about Millie's condition, her upcoming discharge needs, and the conflict between Millie and her daughter about discharge placement). These concerns involve collaborative work with interdisciplinary health care teams to help Millie and her daughter achieve the health goals. With the adaptations made by the project team to Millie's scenario 2, beginning-level QSEN KSAs are reiterated and expanded, while higher-level KSAs are introduced.

The KSA defined for the Safety competency are addressed through Millie's fall. In this scenario, it is noted that a fall-risk assessment was not completed. Millie's fall shows the importance of such KSAs as using effective strategies to reduce risk of patient harm and communicating concerns regarding safety issues.

Patient-centered care is emphasized in the second scenario with the recognition of conflict between Millie and her daughter regarding where Millie will live following discharge. Respecting the patient's wishes and supporting the daughter's involvement in her mother's care are nursing actions that surpass basic respect and sensitivity. These topics require thoughtful communication and conflict resolution skills.

TABLE 6.2

Beginner QSEN Competency Focus, Millie Larsen Scenario 1

QSEN Competency	Knowledge/Skills/Attitudes Emphasized at Beginner Level	Millie Larsen Scenario 1 Learning Activity
Patient-Centered Care	• Integrate understanding of multiple dimensions of patient-centered care: Physical comfort and emotional support • Discuss the principles of effective communication. • Assess levels of physical and emotional comfort • Value seeing health care situations "through patients' eyes" • Recognize personally held attitudes about working with patients form different ethnic, cultural, and social backgrounds	• Assess Millie's preferences and values for health care delivery and individualize her care accordingly. • Explore personal attitudes about aging and cultural diversity. • Utilize primary and secondary resources to validate data. • Review data from Millie's chart and compare to physical assessment findings and patient history. • Utilize communication techniques appropriate to Millie's age and mental status. • Discuss professional boundaries. • Use a cognitively appropriate pain scale to assess physical discomfort. • Assess the potential use and benefit of nonpharmacological interventions. • Perform a falls assessment and recognize the potential for falls related to urinary symptoms. • Plan for frequent assessment to prevent falls. • Include daughter in assessment of home environment safety and self-care ability. • Recognize the cause of Millie's high blood pressure and teach Millie and her daughter strategies for home medication compliance. • Begin to explore safety and feasibility of Millie's return to a home care environment on discharge.

Legal and ethical issues are also intermediate-level KSAs; a phone inquiry by a church member about Millie's condition illustrates compliance with HIPPA regulations. The Teamwork and Collaboration competency is emphasized when physical therapy and occupational therapy expertise is sought to address Millie's mobility and activities of daily living.

ADVANCED QSEN COMPETENCIES

The third scenario was adapted to integrate advanced QSEN competencies. Competencies targeted at the advanced level include Patient-Centered Care, Quality Improvement, Safety, Informatics, and Teamwork and Collaboration. Scenario 3 adaptations incorporate polypharmacy, an interdisciplinary team discharge planning meeting, and a root cause analysis related to Millie's fall.

The integration of polypharmacy in this scenario addresses Safety and Patient-Centered Care. To increase the complexity of the scenario by creating the likelihood of an adverse drug interaction, two drugs were added to Millie's medication list for discharge: zolpidem (Ambien) 10 mg and tramadol (Ultram) 50 mg. This combination of drugs and dosages creates a life-threatening situation for an aging adult.

The complex interaction between the myriad of factors that affect the geriatric patient's health and well-being is illustrated in the discharge planning conflicts that evolve in this scenario. Not only is there concern over the amount of medications that Millie will be taking, her daughter is also concerned over the financial demands for her care, her recent confusion, and the fall she experienced while in the hospital. Millie and her daughter are at odds regarding future living arrangements. Students should recognize the complexity of this situation and recommend and conduct an interdisciplinary team discharge meeting (addressing the competency of Teamwork and Collaboration).

The Center for Disease Control and Prevention (CDC, 2011) estimates that one in every three adults who are 65 or older will experience a fall, and of those who fall, 20 percent to 30 percent will experience moderate to severe injuries. Addressing the underlying cause and prevention of future falls through a root cause analysis (RCA) focuses on the Safety and Quality Improvement competencies. Guidelines to systematically conduct an RCA utilizing a fishbone diagram are provided. Conducting an RCA involves systematically examining the incident and identifying potential human factors and system failures that contributed to the fall. Once the underlying factor is discovered, students are encouraged to brainstorm interventions aimed at improving quality and preventing recurrence of the incident.

CONCLUSION

This overview illustrates how an ACE.S scenario is adapted to incorporate the QSEN competencies. A sample of the QSEN competencies and KSAs are illustrated. Likewise, depending on the quality and safety learning objectives, different competencies and KSAs can be incorporated and simulations adapted accordingly. Debriefing following the simulation is essential to student learning and can likewise be tailored to incorporate guided questions that focus on uncovering the quality and safety knowledge that guided student thinking.

Utilizing the collective wisdom of educators and clinicians, we are challenged to set aside traditional models of education. This is especially significant as it relates to care of the aging adult. Today's nurse educators need to operationalize nursing competencies in education through thoughtful teaching strategies that "deepen the values and attitudes required for quality and safety work" (Cronenwett et al., 2007, p. 130). Simulation is a thoughtful approach to stimulate student thinking and demonstrate the complexities of care for the aging adult.

Adoption of simulation across nursing curricula is a complex challenge for nurse educators (Starkweather & Kardong-Edgren, 2008). Faculty interested in learning strategies for successful integration of simulation into nursing curricula are encouraged to review the online courses of "Curriculum Integration" and "Faculty Development," located on the NLN Simulation Innovation Resources Center (SIRC) website, http://sirc.nln.org/.

References

Barton, A., Armstrong, G., Preheim, G., Gelmon, S. B., & Andrus, L. C. (2009). A national Delphi to determine developmental progression of quality and safety competencies in nursing education. *Nursing Outlook, 57*, 313–322.

Centers for Disease Control and Prevention. (2011). *Home and recreational safety. Falls among older adults: An overview.* Retrieved from http://www.cdc.gov/homeandrecreationalsafety/falls/adultfalls.html

Cronenwett, L., Sherwood, G., Barnsteiner, J., Disch, J., Johnson, J., Mitchell, P., & Warren, J. (2007). Quality and safety education for nurses. *Nursing Outlook, 55*, 122–131. doi:10.1016/j.outlook.2007.02.006

Institute of Medicine (2003). Health professions education: A bridge to quality. Washington, DC: National Academies Press.

Page, J. B., Kowlowitz, V., & Alden, K. R. (2010). Development of a scripted ongoing case study focusing on delirium in older adults. *Journal of Continuing Education in Nursing, 41*, 225–230. doi: 10.3928/00220124-20100423-05

Reese, C. R. (2010). ACES Case #1: Millie Larsen. Developed by the National League for Nursing, Simulation Team Advancing Gerontological Education Strategies (STAGES). Retrieved from www.nln.org/facultydevelopment/facultyresources/aces/millie.htm

Starkweather, A. R., & Kardong-Edgren, S. (2008). Diffusion of innovation: Embedding simulation into nursing curricula. *International Journal of Nursing Education Scholarship, 5*(1), 1–11. Retrieved from http://www.bepress.com

7

ACE.S Program Evaluation: Faculty Use of the ACE.S Concepts and Resources

Eunice S. King, PhD, RN

INTRODUCTION AND BACKGROUND

The Advancing Care Excellence for Seniors (ACE.S) program was designed to provide nursing faculty with the gerontological nursing expertise and teaching resources needed to enhance gerontological nursing content in pre-licensure nursing programs. The need to improve the quality of gerontological nursing content in undergraduate nursing curricula had been documented in work by Berman et al. (2005), Gilje, Lacey, & Moore (2007), and Ironside, Tagliareni, McLaughlin, King, & Mengel (2010). The Ironside et al. study specifically recommended the development of innovative programs to update faculty's gerontological nursing expertise and resources, such as case studies and teaching strategies that could be easily incorporated into lesson plans. The Advancing Care Excellence for Seniors project led by the National League for Nursing was developed and piloted to address this need. (For a comprehensive description of the ACE.S' project development, see Tagliareni, Cline, Mengel, McLaughlin, & King (2012)).

The Integrating Geriatrics into Nursing Education program focused primarily on dissemination of the ACE.S framework and gerontological nursing and teaching resources.

The basic components of the Integrating Geriatrics into Nursing Education program included:

> A one-day faculty workshop. All workshops followed a standard curriculum taught by a team of ACE.S faculty experts utilizing the same content and power points. Between February 2012 and May 2014, 28 workshops were held in 24 different states.

> Two webinars. Webinar 1 was prerecorded and could be viewed at a participant's convenience. Webinar 2, a live webinar, was conducted by the same two ACE.S faculty experts throughout the three-year program period. Didactic material on the use of ACE.S resources and teaching strategies and an update on emerging gerontological content were supplemented by live discussion among webinar participants.

> A one-day workshop held immediately prior to the National League for Nursing's Annual Education Summit (pre-summit workshop) with updates on emergent topics

related to gerontological nursing, presentations on the integration of ACE.S into nursing curriculum, and discussions about the use of ACE.S resources in teaching geriatrics; and

› A website with gerontological nursing education resources including unfolding case studies of older adults with complex health problems, teaching strategies, and links to other websites with resources, such as the Hartford Institute for Geriatric Nursing Resources.

Workshop attendees paid a $100 workshop registration fee that entitled them to participate in both webinars and to attend the pre-NLN Summit workshop. In addition, Continuing Education Units (CEUs) were available for attendance or participation in any of the educational offerings. This chapter reports findings of the evaluation conducted to assess the use of ACE.S and its related resources by faculty ACE.S workshop attendees. The data presented were obtained primarily from an online survey distributed to all faculty workshop attendees one year following their attendance at one of the workshops.

PROGRAM EVALUATION

Although the program evaluation assessed (a) the scope of program dissemination, and (b) the immediate effect of the workshop on the participants' intentions to use ACE.S concepts and resources in their teaching, the focus of this chapter will be on a presentation and discussion of data related to the use of the ACE.S framework concepts and resources. Data for this evaluation came from (a) workshop registrations, (b) website usage statistics about the number of visits to the ACE.S website and views of its pages, and (c) a one-year post-workshop follow-up survey.

ONE-YEAR POST-ACE.S WORKSHOP FOLLOW-UP SURVEY

The one-year follow-up survey of ACE.S workshop attendees was conducted (a) to ascertain the extent to which faculty workshop attendees had used the ACE.S framework concepts and resources introduced during the year post workshop attendance, (b) to find out how they had been used, and (c) to obtain an estimate of the number of nursing students exposed to the ACE.S Framework and resources. It also provided data to describe current faculty respondents' teaching responsibilities and their expertise in gerontological nursing. The survey was conducted between March 2013 and August 2015, ending approximately 15 months after the last workshop was conducted.

Survey Instrument

The survey instrument was comprised of 14 items with subsections that queried respondents about their current faculty responsibilities and expertise in gerontological nursing, their participation in ACE.S educational programs, and their use of ACE.S resources and components of the ACE.S framework. Although many items had been used in prior ACE.S related surveys, the instrument underwent extensive pretesting and multiple revisions to ensure response ease and an average survey completion time of approximately 10 minutes.

Procedures

Response rates to online surveys typically range between a low of 7% to a high of 33%, with the mean hovering around 25% (Penwarden, October 8, 2014). The survey procedures outlined below, considered best practices for improving survey response rates, were utilized to maximize our response rate (Monroe & Adams, 2012; Nulty, 2008; Penwarden, September 25, 2014).

> - During the concluding session of each workshop, the faculty informed the attendees that they would be contacted a year hence and asked to complete a brief survey about their experience using the ACE.S framework and/or the resources. The importance of the survey data in guiding future refinements and expansions to the program was emphasized.
> - One year after attending an ACE.S workshop, Dr. Tagliareni, the NLN program director, sent an email to all attendees notifying them about the upcoming survey and its purposes, and requesting their participation. This enabled the team to identify workshop attendees with undeliverable email addresses and allowed time for project staff to attempt to obtain accurate email addresses.
> - Approximately one week later, the NLN sent an email with the link to the online survey. The email also contained assurances about the confidentiality and anonymity of all responses, the importance of the survey, and information about the incentive for completing the survey—a chance to win a prepaid registration for an NLN Summit being held within the next two years.
> - The survey could be accessed by an attendee for a period of three months. Survey start and completion dates were adjusted slightly to accommodate the academic schedule.
> - Survey completion rates were carefully monitored and email reminders were sent every two to three weeks to nonresponders.

Survey Response Rate

A total of 2128 faculty attended one of the 28 ACE.S workshops conducted between February 2012 and June 2014 and were contacted about participating in the one-year follow-up survey. Of those, 40 were lost to follow-up due to undeliverable email addresses and unavailability of an accurate email address. The denominator on which the response rate was computed was reduced by 40, making it 2088. There were 663 respondents, yielding a response rate of 32%.

Data Analysis

Data from the online survey software were exported into a central database. Univariate statistics were used to analyze responses to all items. Within group analyses using both univariate statistics and cross tabulations, as indicated, were employed to further describe patterns of utilization.

EVALUATION FINDINGS

Workshop Participant Characteristics

These data came exclusively from the 663 individuals who completed the one-year post-ACE.S workshop survey and represented approximately one-third of the actual attendees.

> Of the 663 survey respondents, 96% were actively engaged in the teaching, advisement, and/or supervision of nursing students. As Figure 7.1 shows, the majority were faculty in either an associate degree or baccalaureate nursing program.

> The majority (74%) had obtained their expertise in gerontological nursing through self-directed study that included workshops, seminars, courses, and/or independent study. Only 12% reported having completed a graduate degree, MSN or PhD. with an emphasis in gerontology.

> During the year following the workshop, the majority of respondents (75%) had been responsible for teaching gerontological nursing content.

> Almost half (46%) of the survey respondents indicated that their school or program was actively making changes to enhance the gerontological nursing content in the

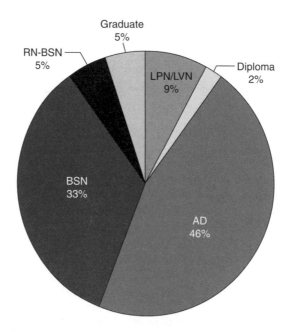

FIGURE 7.1 Type of nursing program in which survey respondents had primary faculty responsibilities.

curriculum. Of the remaining 54%, half described their program as actively discussing ways to enhance the gerontological nursing content in the curriculum.

Commonly Used Resources for Teaching Gerontological Nursing Content

Figure 7.2 shows the resources most respondents used either "sometimes" or "regularly" to guide the selection of gerontological nursing content in the curriculum. Although those with the most frequent regular use were medical surgical nursing textbooks (61%), ACE.S resources had the highest combined "sometimes" and "regular" use.

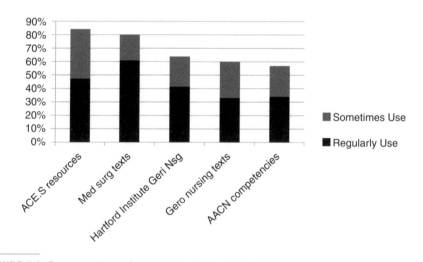

FIGURE 7.2 Frequency of use of resources to guide gerontological nursing content.

ACE.S Resources

During the ACE.S workshops, attendees were introduced to a number of gerontological nursing teaching resources that were readily accessible on the ACE.S website:

1. Links to other online gerontological nursing resources, such as the AJN/ Hartford "How to try this series" or Consult Geri RN;
2. Teaching strategies such as geriatric syndromes, assessment of older adults in long-term care, student-led geriatric nursing conferences, etc.;
3. First-person monologues;
4. Unfolding case studies of older adults; and
5. Instructor toolkits for each of the unfolding case studies.

Of those surveyed, 94% (624) reported having used at least one of the ACE.S resources during the past year. As seen in Figure 7.3, those with the most frequent

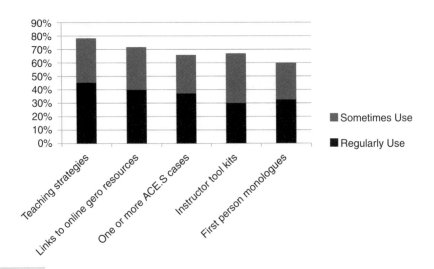

FIGURE 7.3 Frequency of use of ACE.S resources.

regular use were the teaching strategies (45%), followed by links to other online ger-ontological nursing resources (39%), and the unfolding case studies (37%). In addition, 78% (467) reported having used the unfolding case studies at some point during the preceding year. Over the four-year program period (September 2011 through June 2015), the total number of views of the unfolding case studies on the ACE.S website was over 70,000 (70,352) and almost 30,000 (29,970) nursing students were estimated to have been exposed to the ACE.S case studies.

Among the mere 39 faculty who had not used any of the ACE.S resources, the most important reasons for not having done so were the lack of opportunity (59%), lack of relevancy to content taught (49%), or the need to obtain the "buy in" of other faculty. Only 13% cited satisfaction with current resources as an important reason for not using the ACE.S resources. The majority (74%) indicated that it was at least somewhat likely that they would use the ACE.S resources in the future.

Use of the ACE.S Framework

The ACE.S framework guides the care of older adults and is embedded within all of the ACE.S resources. The framework is comprised of three essential knowledge domains—individualized aging, complexity of care, and vulnerability during life transitions—and four essential nursing actions—assess function and expectations, coordinate and manage care, use evolving knowledge, and make situational decisions. The majority of respondents, 79% (484), reported that they had used the ACE.S framework in teaching about the care of older adults, exposing 36,545 students to the knowledge domains and essential nursing actions. As Figure 7.4 shows, the framework had been used in a number of ways, but the three most often cited were (a) to further students' understanding of complexity in caring for older adults, (b) to strengthen the clinical assessment of older adults, and (c) to optimize students' knowledge-based decision making. Among

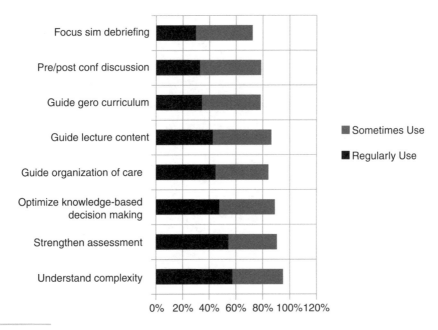

FIGURE 7.4 Use of ACE.S framework components.

the 129 respondents (21%) who had not used the ACE.S framework components, the most important barriers were related to lack of time and opportunity. Eighty-three percent (83%) of those who had not used ACE.S indicated they were at least somewhat likely to use some of the framework components in the future.

OBTAINING FACULTY BUY-IN FOR USE OF THE ACE.S FRAMEWORK AND RESOURCES

For some of the respondents, obtaining the "buy-in" of other faculty posed an important barrier to their use of the ACE.S framework and resources. Twenty-five percent (146) of the respondents noted they had experienced challenges from faculty peers when trying to incorporate the ACE.S concepts and resources. Thirty-seven percent (37%) cited needing to obtain "buy in" from colleagues as a reason for not having used the ACE.S framework components and 44% indicated it prevented them for not having used any of the resources. Of those who had encountered challenges, 97% had attempted to surmount them through use of one or several of the strategies shown in Figure 7.5.

The strategies used most often to obtain the "buy in" of colleagues were to share information about ACE.S and the website resources and/or to introduce ACE.S concepts and resources gradually, using just one or two at a time. Other strategies that had been successful were connecting ACE.S with something of high interest to the faculty, such as simulation, and demonstrating how components of ACE.S or the resources could be used in other courses.

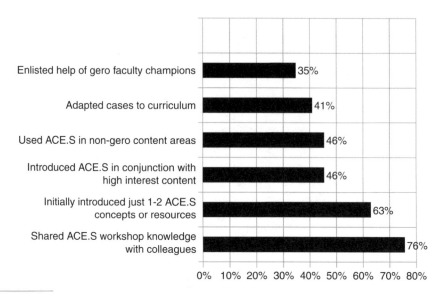

FIGURE 7.5 Strategies used to overcome challenges in incorporating ACE.S concepts and/or resources.

DISCUSSION

Results of this evaluation show that "Integrating geriatrics into nursing education" was very successful in disseminating the ACE.S program widely and in facilitating the use of ACE.S resources and the ACE.S framework by a large number of faculty and nursing programs. One year after attending an ACE.S workshop, 79% of those surveyed reported having used the ACE.S framework concepts, 94% reported having used at least one or more of the ACE.S resources, and 84% had attempted to introduce the ACE.S framework and/or resources into their school or program's curriculum. It is likely that the actual use of ACE.S concepts was closer to 94% or higher, as all of the resources have components of the ACE.S framework embedded within them and, in effect, those who had used the ACE.S resources had also used the framework. The distinction made by two different survey items querying about the use of the resources vs. the ACE.S framework might have confused some respondents. However, since it was possible for faculty to use the ACE.S framework without using any of the ACE.S resources, that item was included to capture the full scope of ACE.S utilization.

One of the most important indicators of the program's success was not only the program participation and subsequent ACE.S utilization, but also, and more impressively, its geographic and program reach. Montana and Alaska were the only states without representation among the attendees at any of the ACE.S workshops. What was particularly notable was the number of nursing programs and/or schools represented by faculty in attendance at the workshops—735 unique nursing programs. In most nursing programs, continuing education workshops, such as this one, are often attended by only one or two faculty, due to budgetary and scheduling issues, and it is expected, and sometimes required, that faculty who attend a workshop share the information with colleagues, either formally or informally. Recall that 76% of these survey respondents reported that they had done just this. Therefore, while the number of workshop attendees is important in disseminating new knowledge, more significant is the number of actual nursing programs represented, as each program represents a potential opportunity for introducing students to ACE.S.

In addition to the high percentage of survey respondents reporting use of ACE.S, another encouraging finding was that they also reported the highest combined "sometimes" and "regular" use of ACE.S resources in guiding the selection of gerontological nursing content in their curriculum. A review and analysis of the gerontological nursing content in five current general medical surgical nursing textbooks, the second most frequently consulted resource, found the gerontological nursing content to be poorly covered and presented (Cline, Manchester, & Tagliareni, 2012). Thus, more frequent use of the ACE.S resources could be an important contributor to improving the quality of pre-licensure gerontological nursing content.

There were many aspects about the ACE.S program implementation that contributed to its success. First, the ACE.S framework and related resources had been carefully developed, as described by Tagliareni, et al. (2012) and the workshops had been pilot tested prior to this program of national dissemination. Second, the program design, the one-day workshop followed by the webinars and access to the ACE.S website to reinforce and expand upon the information, was consistent with how most faculty obtained their knowledge about gerontological nursing—continuing education programs and self-directed study. In addition, for many faculty, this program was very timely. Seventy-three percent (73%) of the faculty surveyed reported that their programs were either actively making changes (46%) to enhance the gerontological nursing content or were actively discussing ways to do so (27%). The ACE.S program provided them with a new approach to teaching about the care of older adults and, very importantly, with rigorously developed and tested resources that could be easily incorporated into their teaching. Approximately one-third of those who completed the online survey took the additional time to add very favorable "optional" comments about the ACE.S program.

LIMITATIONS OF THE EVALUATION

When interpreting the results of this evaluation, the reader is reminded that data related to use of the ACE.S framework and resources, came from an online survey of approximately 32% of the ACE.S workshop participants. Although this response rate is in the upper range for online surveys, it does represent slightly less than one-third of the actual workshop attendees, thereby raising potential threats to the validity of the findings. The two outcomes for which this is potentially an issue in this evaluation are the post-workshop utilization rates of the ACE.S framework components and ACE.S resources, respectively. It can be argued that the high utilization rates reported might be due to a self-selection sample bias, such that those who participated in the survey were those who were more interested in ACE.S than those who did not. Potential sample bias for other survey items related to how the ACE.S resources and framework were used are not subject to the same validity concerns as that information pertains only to ACE.S users.

If one were to assume that all of those workshop attendees who did not complete the survey had also not used ACE.S (a very unlikely scenario), and to compute an overall

ACE.S' use rate with ACE.S resource use as the indicator, a very conservative estimate of ACE.S utilization during the year following the ACE.S workshop for all attendees would be 30% (i.e., 624/2088). A 30% adoption rate of an innovation by individuals within the first year of its introduction is commendable. Then, when one computes an ACE.S adoption rate by school/ program, that rate is even more impressive, as it gives a more accurate picture of the scope of ACE.S dissemination. The 624 survey respondents indicating use of ACE.S represented 353 of the 735 distinct schools or programs with attendees at the workshops. Thus, almost half (48%) of the schools/programs represented at the ACE.S workshops used ACE.S within the following year, exposing a total of 36,545 students to the ACE.S framework and 29,970 to the unfolding case studies.

FUTURE DIRECTIONS

There is no question that this program was successful in assisting many pre-licensure nursing programs with their efforts to enhance the quality of gerontological nursing education. However, there are at least two challenges to be addressed in the future. The first is to address questions about how students exposed to ACE.S use this approach as graduate nurses caring for older adults and how the use of ACE.S affects the health outcomes for older adults. An analysis of each of the three major concepts underlying the ACE.S framework—complexity, individual aging, and vulnerability during transitions—will provide researchers with definitions of each concept that can facilitate the design of studies to address these questions (Cline, 2014, 2015, 2016).

The second challenge is to support faculty's continued interest in using ACE.S and to disseminate ACE.S further. Implementing change is often met with resistance, as noted by many survey respondents who reported the necessity of obtaining the buy in of other faculty and of receiving support for their efforts. The "Integrating Geriatrics into Nursing Education" program provided faculty support through discussions at the pre-summit workshops and during Webinar 2. However, once the ACE.S dissemination program concluded, strategies for supporting faculty's continued interest in using ACE.S and disseminating ACE.S further have remained to be addressed. One such strategy is ACESXPRESS, a microsite of the ACE.S website (www.nln.org/ACESXPRESS), a digital campaign developed during the fourth year of this program to address these challenges and to continue to introduce new free ACE.S resources for implementing best practices in gerontology. On this site are a library of short videos, ranging in length from 90 seconds to 4 minutes, archived webinars, twitter chats, and links to other ACE.S resources. Additionally, the NLN has developed strategic partnerships with key national organizations (e.g., AARP, NSNA, and the Hartford Institute at NYU) to increase social media exposure for ACESXPRESS. During the nine months following the campaign launch in late January 2015, there were 6,533 sessions tracked and 5,259 new site-users, underscoring the potential efficacy of this strategy for continued use and dissemination of ACE.S.

Finally, several of the ACE.S workshop attendees requested that the ACE.S framework be applied to the care of other populations as well. Within the past couple of years, the NLN has expanded the application of ACE.S from care of the older adult to care of vulnerable populations and has developed case studies that apply the ACE.S framework to the care of veterans and clients with Alzheimer's disease. The potential for using the ACE.S model in caring for a wide range of vulnerable clients is very exciting.

ACKNOWLEDGMENT

Support for this evaluation was provided by the Independence Foundation. Special thanks go to the following individuals who were most diligent in assisting with data collection and management for this evaluation: Naomi Wetmore, former data and grants manager, Community College of Philadelphia, and Tatiana Nin, ACE.S grant program manager, the National League for Nursing. In addition, the author wishes to thank the ACE.S program leadership team, Dr. Elaine Tagliareni, Chief Program Officer for the NLN, Dr. Andrea Mengel, retired Professor and Independence Foundation Chair, Community College of Philadelphia, and Dr. Barbara McLaughlin, Head, Department of Nursing, Community College of Philadelphia, as well as Dr. Kathy Kaufman for the online survey programming and administration and Ms. Jane Grosset for the data analysis.

References

Berman, A., Mezey, M., Kobayashi, M., Fulmer, T., Stanley, J., & Thornlow, D. (2005). Gerontological nursing content in baccalaureate nursing programs: Comparison of findings from 1997 and 2003. *Journal of Professional Nursing, 21*, 268–275.

Cline, D. D. (2014). A concept analysis of individualized aging. *Nursing Education Perspectives, 35*, 185–191.

Cline, D. D. (2015) Complexity of care: A concept analysis of older adults' health care experiences. *Nursing Education Perspectives, 36*, 108–113.

Cline, D. D. (2016). A concept analysis of vulnerability during transitions. *Nursing Education Perspectives, 37*(2), 91–96.

Cline, D. D., Manchester, J., & Tagliareni, M. E. (2012). Gerontological nursing content in general medical/surgical textbooks: Where is it? *Nursing Education Perspectives, 33*, 150–155.

Gilje, F., Lacey, L., & Moore, C. (2007). Gerontology and geriatric issues and trends in U.S. nursing programs: A national survey. *Journal of Professional Nursing, 23*, 21–29.

Ironside, P., Tagliareni, M., McLaughlin, B., King, E., & Mengel, A. (2010). Fostering geriatrics in associate degree nursing education: An assessment of current curricula and clinical experiences. *Journal of Nursing Education, 49*, 246–252.

Monroe, M., and Adams, D. (2012). Increasing response rates to web-based surveys. *Journal of Extension* [online], *50*(6) Article 6TOT7. Available at http://www.joe.org/joe/2012december.

Nulty, D. (2008). The adequacy of response rates to online and paper surveys: what can be done? [electronic version] *Assessment & Evaluation in Higher Education, 33*, 301–314.

Penwarden, R. (2014, September 25). What is the difference between a response rate and a completion rate? Posted to Fluid Surveys http://fluidsurveys.com/university.

Penwarden, R. (2014, October 8). Response rate statistics for online surveys—What numbers should you be aiming for? Posted to Fluid Surveys http://fluidsurveys.com/university.

Survey response rates: Tips on how to increase your survey response rates. (nd). Retrieved October 2013 from http://peoplepulse.com/resources/useful-articles.

Tagliareni, M., Cline, D., Mengel, A., McLaughlin, B., & King, E. (2012). Quality care for older adults: The NLN advancing care excellence for seniors (ACES) project. *Nursing Education Perspectives, 33*, 144–149.

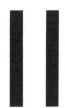

Application of ACE.S: Teaching and Research

This section presents exemplars of how faculty—many of whom are NLN Hearst Foundations Award winners—applied the ACE.S framework to their unique curricula. Chapters 9 and 14 highlight research studies using the ACE.S cases to build student competence in caring for older adults and their caregivers.

8

ACE.S Teaching Resources for Classroom, Simulation and Clinical Practice

M. Elaine Tagliareni, EdD, RN, CNE, FAAN

Mary Anne Rizzolo, EdD, RN, FAAN, ANEF

Laureen Tavolaro-Ryley, MSN, RN, CNS

Tamika Curry, MSN, RN

The NLN ACE.S project is a targeted effort to enhance the geriatric expertise of nursing faculty by providing ACE.S resources and assisting faculty, through workshops and accessible tools on the NLN website, to incorporate them into classroom, skills lab, simulation and clinical nursing experiences. The ultimate goal of ACE.S is to enhance students' learning experiences and prepare nursing graduates to address the complex health care needs of the aging population.

DEVELOPMENT OF ACE.S TEACHING RESOURCES

When the ACE.S project was first conceptualized in 2009, project staff believed firmly that what was needed to fully integrate gerontology into nursing programs nationally was to provide a way for students to learn about care of older adults and to provide tools for nursing faculty to teach students how to care for older adults. Over time, foundational concepts were developed, resulting in the ACE.S Essential Knowledge Domains and Essential Nursing Actions, leading to a strong emphasis on coordinating care during life transitions and recognizing that older adults are our most complex patients, ideas that are fundamental to providing competent, individualized, and humanistic care.

Project staff recognized that adoption and use of the ACE.S Essential Knowledge Domains and Essential Nursing Actions, and true integration of gerontology concepts across the curriculum required us to create teacher-ready, modifiable tools for overburdened faculty. The intent was to assist faculty to work with students to develop nursing judgment, to notice what is happening by assessing the person's functional status along with the strengths, resources, needs, cultural traditions, wishes, and expectations of the older adult and caregiver. The teacher and student would use evolving evidence-based gerontological knowledge, technology, and best practices to encourage a spirit of inquiry, foster evidence-based decision-making, and provide competent care for the older adult and caregiver. The basis of all ACE.S resources would be the ACE.S Knowledge Domains and Essential Nursing Actions, which enable nursing students and practicing nurses to translate their knowledge of individualized aging, complexity of care, and vulnerability during life transitions into actions that promote high-quality care for older adults.

The belief that it is essential that management of chronic care for older adults be more than a series of discrete services was a consistent curriculum focus during development of the resources. Additionally, since a common occurrence for older adults is to move across care settings and experience changes in environment and levels of independence and functioning, incorporation of these dynamic events was deemed essential to include in development of the teaching resources. Another important concept was to create teaching tools for students to use nursing judgment and situational decision making to observe, interpret, respond, and reflect, based on the nurse's knowledge and the older adult or caregiver's expectations. Also, recognizing that adding new content to an already full nursing curriculum is challenging, ACE.S was designed to work without adding additional content. Instead, the idea is to provide modifiable, classroom-ready teaching tools, strategies, and opportunities for interactive learning in a wide variety of settings, from the classroom to acute-care environments, to community-based direct patient care experiences, using common medical conditions that are universally taught (e.g., diabetes, COPD).

The ACE.S staff also recognized the benefits to creating synergy between the ACE.S initiative and other existing gerontological resources, specifically the Hartford-funded organizations and programs, such as *Try This*®, (ConsultGeriRN.org), and geriatric nursing competencies. Finally, project staff felt strongly that teaching strategies needed to focus students to consider the unique needs of older adults and their caregivers, and develop a positive view of aging. The tools needed to be interactive and patient/client centered and address these essential and underlying questions:

▸ How would the teaching of nursing be "turned upside down" if we framed learning activities differently, encouraging students to recognize, respect and respond to the complex nature of care for older adults from the beginning of the nursing program?

▸ How would a significant focus on older adults and their families during life transitions impact situational decision-making by students to manage care in the context of the older adult's needs, wishes, and quality of life?

▸ How would we develop resources to teach students to value assessment of function, expectations and culture when caring for older adults with physical and mental diagnoses?

Eventually, two sets of teaching resources were developed: unfolding cases and teaching strategies. Both the unfolding cases and teaching strategies, provided free on the NLN website, provide realistic encounters with older adults that are intentional and incorporate all or some of the ACE.S Essential Knowledge Domains and Essential Nursing Actions.

ACE.S UNFOLDING CASES

Background

So often students meet an older adult as a one-time event in the acute clinical environment or in a home-care situation. But the lives of older adults are so much more complex. Project staff asked, "How can we assist students to know the richness of the older adult's experiences? Without that knowledge, is individualized care possible?" "How will we teach students about the vulnerability of older adults and their caregivers during transitions and the complex nature of decision-making in those situations?"

Project staff felt that a case study approach was needed, but realized that traditional case studies were based primarily on medical diagnoses and only presented a record of signs and symptoms and a list of demographics describing the patient. This type of presentation would not paint a picture of the uniqueness of the older adult and present a glimpse into the older adult's expectations, wishes, and interpretation of significant life events leading to the current encounter. All of these factors are needed to develop a realistic and individualized plan of care. Therefore, unfolding case studies, beginning with a first-person monologue, with simulation scenarios embedded to provide a picture over time, were developed to create a realistic picture of the health care journey experienced by older adults and their caregivers. This approach, built on narrative pedagogy, had the potential to tell the story from the client's point of view and give the student an understanding that would help them notice and respond to an older adult's functional status, wishes and beliefs. It also provided a unique platform allowing students to feel more connected to the older adults they encountered and more invested in discussing and experiencing their journey with them.

Essential Components

An unfolding case is defined as one that evolves over time in a manner that is unpredictable to the learner. Patient profiles are purposely complicated—like real people. Teaching through case study is widely regarded as an effective teaching methodology when compared with the traditional style of lectures in promoting a learner's critical reasoning skills. The ACE.S unfolding case scenarios combine the power of storytelling with the experiential nature of simulation and provide a simulated experience of continuity of care that is difficult to provide to all students in typical clinical facilities.

The unfolding cases represent a range of challenges faced by older adults, including medical, functional, psychosocial, interpersonal, and financial issues. Four unfolding case study simulation scenarios using the "gero" lens (Millie Larson, Sherman "Red" Yoder, Henry and Ertha Williams, and Julie Morales and Lucy Grey), three Alzheimer's Disease-centered unfolding cases (George Palo, Judy and Karen Jones, and Ertha Williams), and two veterans cases (Butch Sampson and Eugene Shaw) are available on the NLN website (nln.org/ACE). See Box 8.1.

BOX 8.1

Unfolding Cases

Original ACE.S Cases

Millie Larsen: Millie Larson is an 84-year-old widow who lives alone. Her current medical problems include hypertension, glaucoma, osteoarthritis of the knee, stress incontinence, osteoporosis, and hypercholesterolemia.

Red Yoder: Red Yoder is an 80-year-old farmer who lives alone in a farmhouse 20 miles outside of town. Red has been a widower for 10 years. He has insulin-dependent diabetes, some incontinence, and difficulty sleeping. He developed a blister from new shoes which has become infected.

Henry and Ertha Williams is a 69-year-old African American, a retired rail system engineer who lives in a small apartment with his wife, Ertha. Henry and Ertha had one son who was killed in the war 10 years ago. Henry has COPD and he is concerned about Ertha, who has been experiencing frequent memory lapses.

Julia Morales and Lucy Grey: Julia Morales, age 65, and Lucy Grey, age 73, are partners who have been together for more than 25 years. Julia has lung cancer that is no longer responding to chemotherapy and she wants to stop treatment. Lucy is supportive and believes she will be able to care for Julia in their home.

ACE.Z (Alzheimers Disease and their Caregivers) Cases

Ertha Williams: (The ACE.S case of Henry Williams provided an opportunity to continue the journey of Henry and Ertha.) Ertha is 74 years old. She and her husband Henry recently moved to an assisted living facility. Shortly after the move, Henry passed away and Ertha's memory lapses increased. The case unfolds as Ertha is challenged by multiple transitions and subsequent progressive neurocognitive impairment.

George Palo: George Palo is a 90-year-old widower who has been diagnosed with early stage dementia. George is very independent and loves to be outdoors, walking his golden retriever, Max. His daughter, Maggie, and her siblings are trying to support their dad's independence as long as possible, but are cognizant of his age and concerned about his overall safety.

Judy and Karen Jones: Judy Jones is an 85-year-old widow diagnosed with mild dementia. Her oldest daughter, Karen, moved back into the family home to provide support for her mother. Judy is able to stay home alone during the day while Karen is at work.

ACE.V (Advancing Care Excellence for Veterans) Cases

Two of the patients in the ACE.V unfolding cases are older adults. While the primary focus is on recognizing and improving heath care of veterans, they can also be used to reinforce tenets of the ACE.S framework.

Butch Sampson: Butch Sampson, age 62, was exposed to Agent Orange during his service in Vietnam. Chronically homeless, Butch has Type 2 diabetes resulting in the removal of two toes. During the first two simulations, Butch is in a Veterans Administration hospital for surgical debridement of his great toe. He is discharged to a temporary housing facility, but during a visit by the home health nurse, we find that Butch is in danger of being evicted because he has been smoking in his apartment, a violation of the rules.

Eugene Shaw: Gene Shaw, age 82, is a former marine who has had cold sensitization and nocturnal pain in his lower limbs and hands since trench foot, acquired during his service in Korea, required amputation of several toes. He also has hypertension, osteoarthritis, and Type 2 Diabetes. He is overweight, smokes, and drinks. Chronic leg pain and ulcerations lead to a hospital admission for femoral-popliteal by-pass surgery. The nurses who care for Gene must provide emotional support and teaching, and consider changes in life style that may affect his recovery and rehabilitation.

To access the unfolding cases and teaching strategies, go to http://www.nln.org/centers-for-nursing-education/nln-center-for-excellence-in-the-care-of-vulnerable-populations and follow the links.

Cases are written so that they can be modified to meet the needs of diverse curricula, different teaching methods, and individual style. Each case includes the following:

> **A first-person monologue** that introduces the individual or couple and the complex problems to be addressed. The monologue, delivered in the first person, is an audio recording of the person or family member telling their story and setting the stage for the first encounter. The monologues are used by faculty to engage students in a conversation, using principles of active learning. Symptoms are presented in the context of the client's life, and the individual's unique strengths are provided so students can better plan their approaches to care. Factors such as the client's expectations, the risk vs. the benefits of interventions, and functional status are also highlighted to prompt the student to look beyond a set of symptoms and laboratory values.

> **Simulation scenarios** designed to help students practice assessing function and expectations of their patients, then intervene and see the results of their care, provide the core of the unfolding cases. Since good assessment skills are the foundation for appropriate care of older adults, key components of each simulation are the evidence-based assessment tools from the *Try This®: Best Practices in Nursing Care to Older Adults* series. The tools were a John A. Hartford Foundation-funded initiative provided to the Hartford Institute for Geriatric Nursing at New York University's College of Nursing. Collaboration with the American Journal of Nursing (AJN) provided the addition of a *How to Try This®* series, consisting of demonstration videos and a corresponding print series featured in the AJN that effectively translates the evidence-based geriatric assessment tools in the *Try This®* assessment series into cost-free, web-based resources. The extensive and continually expanding resource, found at http://www.consultgerirn.org, provides knowledge of best practices in the care of older adults that is easily accessible, easily understood, easily implemented. The goal is to encourage the use of these best practices by all direct-care nurses.

> **A "finish the story" assignment** that encourages creativity while providing a way to evaluate student's understanding of ACE.S concepts. Some students have written scholarly papers and created alternative endings and additional simulation scenarios, while others have written poems and songs that reflect empathy, caring, and a deep understanding of what it means to be an older adult who is experiencing multiple health care problems and difficult transitions. It is an opportunity for students to again look beyond concrete symptoms, and think in a more thoughtful way about outcomes of care.

> **An instructor toolkit** with suggestions on how to use the various components of the unfolding cases provides additional and essential assistance to overburdened faculty so they can easily adopt the unfolding cases and incorporate them into the curriculum.

TEACHING STRATEGIES

The NLN ACE.S project provides teaching strategies that are guides for faculty to develop encounters with older adults that incorporate all or some of the ACE.S Essential Knowledge Domains and Essential Nursing Actions. The template for the teaching strategies includes: an overview, learning objectives, ideas to "get started", materials (e.g., PowerPoint slides, concept map templates, suggested reflection questions) and optional readings for students with references.

Teaching strategies are available to download for use in any course. Examples include:

▸ *Utilizing Resources to Support Independence and Quality of Life Issues in Older Adults:* Feeling productive, relevant, and independent are significant to older adults. This teaching strategy focuses on working collaboratively with an older adult who has both physical and psychosocial challenges to find resources to maintain independence and strategize to optimize his quality of life.

▸ *Mental Health Needs of Older Adults:* Managing multiple conditions, including atypical presentations of diseases, in both daily life and during life transitions is complex. This strategy highlights issues integral to patients and families.

▸ *Dorothy as the Prototype in Looking at Client Expectations; Quality of Life and Functioning:* Maximizing functional status and maintaining independence in light of multiple co-morbidities makes care multifaceted. This is a key understanding from this teaching strategy using the Dorothy monologue.

▸ *Elder Abuse in the United States:* Advocacy is a major role for the nurse. The nurse needs to advocate and provide comprehensive care during acute exacerbations of chronic conditions, and address the continuing chronic care needs simultaneously. This is a key understanding in this teaching strategy.

▸ *Using the Monologue of Doris Smith to Understand Situational Decision-Making:* Nurses often find themselves wondering if the care decisions they make produce the best outcomes for older adults. This teaching strategy addresses the need for effective situational decision making.

▸ *Assessment of Older Adults in Long-Term Care:* Through planned, intentional encounters with older adults, nursing students learn to promote human flourishing and to provide competent, individualized, and humanistic care. This teaching strategy focuses on assessment in long-term care clinical settings with students in both beginning and advanced nursing courses.

▸ *End-of-Life Decision Making for Older Adults: Competent and Compassionate Care: Geriatric Syndromes:* Understanding new knowledge, especially new evidence about geriatric syndromes and unique presentations of common symptoms in older adults is essential during this vulnerable period.

▸ *Examining Risks and Benefits to Enhance Quality of Life:* Helping older adults and their care-givers to make situational decisions about nursing care based on the older adult's wishes as well as the overall treatment plan. This is seen in the Doris teaching strategy and the teaching strategy about examining risks and benefits (under individualized care). This teaching strategy assists students to examine their own beliefs about how to weigh risks and benefits.

▸ *Caring for the Caregiver:* Helping caregivers to feel more secure in the caregiving role is an essential nursing role. Supporting them during the often turbulent transitions between care settings can help with more favorable outcomes for them as well as the patient as indicated by this teaching strategy.

New teaching strategies are continually being updated, extended, and revised and will continue to be released by the NLN; NLN members are alerted when new resources are made available on the NLN ACE.S's website.

ACESXPRESS

In January 2015, the NLN launched ACESXPRESS, a digital campaign to build a wider audience for use of ACE.S free resources. As part of the campaign, the NLN developed four videos to explain the ACE.S story, provide an overview of the ACE.S Essential Knowledge Domains and Essential Nursing Actions, and deliver a message from NLN CEO, Dr. Beverly Malone, inviting nursing students to take on the challenge and the joy of a career working with older adults and their caregivers (http://www.nln.org/acesxpress/). The website also includes starter kits that provide selected unfolding cases and teaching strategies targeted to mental health needs, caregiving special considerations, individualized aging, complexity of care and vulnerability during life transitions. In this way, faculty can access the starter kits to plan curricula directed to specific topics. Through ACESXPRESS, the NLN and its strategic partners seek to foster a rich ongoing conversation among a diverse community of educators invested in improving care for this vulnerable population.

CONCLUSION

The chapters that follow this overview of NLN ACE.S teaching resources describe ways faculty have applied the ACE.S unfolding cases and teaching strategies, both to conduct research and to tailor them to meet course and program objectives. Nursing must be at the forefront of improving care of older adults. By advancing the cause, and providing an adaptable, classroom-ready and comprehensive educational approach—the NLN ACE.S project gives nurse educators and students alike a way to provide individualized, and high-quality care to older adults and their caregivers.

9

Enhancing Clinical Reasoning Through Simulation Debriefing: A Multisite Study

Susan G. Forneris, PhD, RN, CNE, CHSE-A
Diana Odland Neal, PhD, RN
Jone Tiffany, DNP, RN, RNC
Mary Beth Kuehn, EdD, RN, PHN
Heidi M. Meyer, MSN, RN, PHN
Linda M. Blazovich, DNP, RN, CNE
Ann E. Holland, PhD, RN
Melanie Smerillo, MSN, RN, PHN

ABSTRACT

AIM: The aim of this research was to replicate Dreifuerst's 2012 findings of enhanced clinical reasoning scores using a structured debriefing: Debriefing for Meaningful Learning© (DML).

BACKGROUND: The direct effect of debriefing on clinical reasoning is not well studied. The nursing education literature supports debriefing as a reflective dialogue necessary to enhance clinical reasoning.

METHOD: A quasi-experimental, pre-test–post-test, repeated measure research design was used to evaluate nursing students' clinical reasoning using the Health Sciences Reasoning Test (HSRT).

RESULTS: The change in HSRT mean scores was determined to be significant for the intervention group at the .05 level and insignificant for the control group. The change in HSRT mean scores between the intervention and control groups was determined to be significant at the .10 level.

CONCLUSION: Nursing students who had the DML debriefing scored significantly higher in their clinical reasoning than nursing students who had usual and customary debriefing.

With a focus on developing sound critical thinking and clinical reasoning skills, the goal of contemporary nursing education is to teach students to think like a nurse (Tanner, 2006). Thus, nurse educators seek to engage students in thinking that goes beyond the boundaries of memorization and struggle to demonstrate the effectiveness of teaching strategies that have a positive impact on critical thinking and clinical reasoning (Forneris & Peden-McAlpine, 2007).

For the past 10 years, simulation and debriefing have gained momentum as active teaching-learning strategies that successfully impact student thinking along the learning continuum (Jeffries, 2012). Debriefing for Meaningful Learning© (DML) is a method of structured reflective debriefing developed by Dreifuerst (2009) that has been studied in simulation research, with significant findings for positive changes in clinical reasoning (Dreifuerst, 2012; Mariani, Cantrell, Meakim, Prieto, & Dreifuerst, 2013). This article reports findings from a nursing education simulation study intended to replicate Dreifuerst's findings regarding the impact of DML on clinical reasoning across multiple sites.

BACKGROUND

The use of simulation in nursing education provides opportunities to practice clinical reasoning skills in a controlled environment (Jeffries, 2012). Debriefing is a key component of simulation and its importance is well documented in the literature (Cantrell, 2008; Fanning & Gaba, 2007; Neill & Wotton, 2011; Shinnick, Woo, Horwich, & Steadman, 2011). Debriefing skills are highly variable and dependent upon faculty preparation and training. Competence in debriefing is considered as important in simulation as the skill required to write and develop simulation scenarios or the programming of high-fidelity simulators (Jeffries, 2005). Jeffries (2005) discusses a theoretical framework for simulation and debriefing that is influenced, in part, by sound educational practices. These practices, which include principles of active learning, feedback, and collaboration, provide structure to effective debriefing and ultimately influence student learning outcomes.

The direct effect of simulation and debriefing on learner performance and clinical reasoning is not well studied. Only a few research studies have examined the effectiveness of debriefing to enhance learner performance (Cicero et al., 2012; Kuiper, Heinrich, Matthias, Graham, & Bell-Kotwell, 2008; Shinnick et al., 2011). In recent years, reflective debriefing practices to specifically enhance clinical reasoning have been developed. These practices engage learners in critical conversations to uncover the thinking behind actions performed during simulation (Dreifuerst, 2009).

Engaging learners in critical conversations using higher level questioning is not a new strategy (Forneris, 2004; Forneris & Peden-McAlpine, 2006, 2007; Myrick & Yonge, 2002, 2003), and engaging critical conversations in debriefing of simulation has become more popular. Debriefing provides an opportunity to reframe the use of reflection and dialogue through a learner-centered approach that guides thinking and helps the learner make an inferential link between thinking and doing (Decker, 2007; Dreifuerst, 2009; Jeffries, 2012; Lasater, 2007; Parker & Myrick, 2010). Thus, debriefing has become a catalyst in assisting nurse educators to teach clinical reasoning skills.

Gaining in popularity, Dreifuerst's DML is structured to guide learners through a process of reflecting on and explaining their thinking within the context of their experience, making known the reasoning and knowledge behind their actions (2009). This connection between thinking and doing fosters new understanding that can then be transferred to new practice experiences (Schön, 1983, 1987).

REVIEW OF THE LITERATURE

The opportunities that simulation provides to practice clinical reasoning skills in a controlled environment are highlighted in the literature (Jeffries, 2012). Debriefing as a component of simulation is the ability to engage learners through the use of reflection and dialogue to enhance clinical reasoning (Decker, 2007; Dreifuerst, 2009; Jeffries; Lasater, 2007). Only a few studies have specifically studied the use of structured debriefing to achieve measurable changes in student learning and behavior.

Structured Debriefing to Improve Student Performance

Kuiper et al. (2008) used the Outcome Present State-Test Model (OPT), a structured debriefing activity utilizing clinical reasoning during high-fidelity simulation. The constructivist learning theory underpinning this debriefing approach suggests that the situated cognition and reasoning skills used to solve the problems encountered in simulation are comparable to the experiences and reasoning skills used in authentic clinical environments. The goal of the study was to compare simulated clinical experiences with authentic experiences and, specifically, learners' situated cognition using OPT to determine if the OPT model could be used as a method of debriefing.

The OPT model to structure debriefing uses organization, comparison, classification, evaluation, summarization, and analysis and is operationalized using a specific worksheet following debriefing with faculty. Forty-four students participated in both high-fidelity simulations and authentic clinical experiences; no significant difference was found in OPT scores. Kuiper et al. (2008) suggest that the OPT model and the use of OPT worksheets can provide the reflection and scaffolding needed in both simulation and authentic practice.

Pediatric disaster medicine (PDM) triage skills were studied during a multipatient simulation followed by a structured debriefing (Cicero et al., 2012). Structured debriefing was defined as a process of formative evaluation that involved the learner in a reflective process comparing the current educational experience to a prior experience with a closing conversation targeted toward future improvement of performance. Fifty-three students took part in pediatric disaster simulations. Following each simulation, structured debriefing took place with a discussion on triage rationale. The students were involved in new simulations one week later and again five weeks later; triage accuracy improved by the third round of simulation and structured debriefing.

Structured Debriefing to Improve Clinical Reasoning

Debriefing for Meaningful Learning is grounded in the work of Schön (1983) and utilizes a consistent process to guide student reflection and dialogue throughout the learning experience. The learner is guided through a reflective conversation to discern what is relevant and meaningful, given the context of a situation. Dreifuerst (2012) incorporates six essential components to assist faculty in a guided process to engage, explore, explain, elaborate, evaluate, and extend the thinking of learners (Bybee et al., 1989). Through this active learning process, the learner reflects on the practice situation based on current knowledge and constructs new or revised meaning based on experiential learning (Kolb, 1984). The DML provides an opportunity for students to analyze action, uncover rationale, and direct future action (Dreifuerst, 2012). In developing her approach to debriefing, Dreifuerst focused specifically on the use of debriefing to enhance clinical reasoning skills. The DML process helps learners reflect on their nursing knowledge from different perspectives, transform to new understanding, and improve their process of thinking (Dreifuerst, 2009).

Dreifuerst (2012) used the Health Sciences Reasoning Test (HSRT) to study the relationship between the DML process and the development of clinical reasoning skills in 238 pre-licensure nursing students following high-fidelity adult health simulations. The HSRT was used for both pre-test and post-test. Students who were debriefed using the DML process had higher overall HSRT post-test scores than students who were debriefed with usual and customary methods. A positive relationship was found between the DML as a debriefing method and clinical reasoning skill development.

Mariani et al. (2013) used the Lasater Clinical Judgment Rubric (LCJR) (Lasater, 2007) to study the effect of the DML on clinical judgment with 86 junior nursing students during the first semester of a junior-level medical-surgical nursing course. Students involved in the study participated in two simulations, one at midterm and the other at the end of the semester; the DML was used for the intervention group. Clinical judgment was assessed using the LCJR at the conclusion of each simulation.

The intervention group yielded higher clinical judgment scores than the control group; however, the differences were not statistically significant. Students perceived that the DML enhanced student-focused learning in contrast to the customary debriefing, which was more teacher centered.

These studies inform our understanding of the effectiveness of simulation and debriefing on student learning, but they are single-site studies. The NLN, in its *Research Priorities in Nursing Education* (2012), calls for robust research designs through the use of multisite approaches. A second priority is to evaluate the effectiveness of creative teaching-learning methodologies, such as simulation and debriefing, to enhance clinical reasoning skills. Adamson, Kardong-Edgren, and Willhaus (2013) call for pedagogies that move students toward changes in behaviors that improve patient care outcomes. They note that further study and evaluation are warranted to duplicate findings in different populations. This article reports the findings of a multisite study that replicates Dreifuerst's single-site study (2012) to investigate the impact of the DML on clinical reasoning. Two research questions were asked:

> ▸ Does the use of the DML debriefing method positively impact the development of clinical reasoning skills in undergraduate nursing students compared to usual and customary debriefing?

> ▸ Do nursing students perceive a difference in the quality of debriefing when the DML method is used compared to usual and customary debriefing?

METHOD

This study was conducted at four baccalaureate colleges of nursing in the Midwest. A pilot study was conducted the year prior to ensure consistency with research methods, procedures, and instruments. All the student groups involved in the pilot and main studies were enrolled full-time in their respective baccalaureate nursing programs. All four baccalaureate programs were part of nursing departments of faith-based private colleges. The student groups in the main study were determined to be homogenous.

A quasi-experimental, pre-test/post-test, repeated measure research design was used to answer the research questions. A convenience sample of 200 nursing students at the beginning of their second year of course work (seniors) was the purposive, target population. To obtain a medium effect size of .50 and 80 percent power, 200 participants were estimated to be necessary a priori according to Lipsey (1990) and confirmed using G-Power analysis (Faul, Erdfelder, Buchner, & Lang, 2009). The study was approved by the institutional review board of each college/university. Students were informed verbally and in writing about the research study and provided their consent.

Sample

Of the 200 eligible nursing students, 156 senior students enrolled in the study; 153 fully participated. Of the participating students, 78 were randomly assigned to the intervention group (DML debriefing) and 75 to the control group (usual and customary debriefing). All students completed the simulation experience at their home institutions in familiar simulation labs. To assure that students would not be disadvantaged, the DML debriefing method was incorporated into all students' simulation course work after post-testing was completed.

Procedure

The NLN's Advancing Care Excellence for Seniors (ACE.S) Millie Larsen geriatric simulation scenario was selected as the simulation experience. Millie Larsen (Reese, 2010) is an unfolding three-scenario simulation featuring a geriatric patient experiencing complications from dehydration, a urinary tract infection, and a complex transition process. The case was adapted to include a patient fall and polypharmacy issues. The ACE.S scenario was chosen because it features common content across the four campus nursing programs for completion of aging, adult health, and medical-surgical content areas.

Participants completed the Health Sciences Reasoning Test (HSRT) during their first week of classes. Prior to participating in a simulation, students completed preparation materials outlining objectives, performance expectations, and preparatory activities (e.g., creation of medication cards, reviewing diagnosis, describing pathophysiology, completing readings and resource materials, anticipating potential complications). After they participated in the ACE.S simulation lab and subsequent debriefing, they completed the DASH©-SV evaluation of their simulation experience. Three weeks later, they completed a second version of the HSRT.

As in Dreifuerst's study, participants took an alternate post-test version of the HSRT, which was similar but not identical to the first to eliminate bias due to familiarity with the items. A period of at least two weeks is recommended between pre-test and post-test to avoid a familiarity effect whereby students choose answers on the post-test based on something they remember from the pre-test (Facione & Facione, 2006).

The simulation lab consisted of three 20-minute unfolding simulation scenarios, each followed by a separate debriefing. To ensure consistency in procedures across the multiple sites, preparation of the labs, props and supplies, and medical records were matched across campuses. Each scenario was specifically scripted to ensure reliability of student cueing and consistency for standardized patient (SP) performance.

Each campus recruited nursing alumni and/or community members to perform the SP roles of the patient and family member. Prior to the role-playing, the SP received training on the written scenario progression and cueing. Each unfolding scenario was followed by a 40-minute debriefing session using the DML or a 20-minute usual and customary debriefing. Each debriefing style had a standard set of learning outcomes and talking points or guided questions.

Four research team members were trained in DML methodology and were assigned to debrief intervention groups outside their home campuses. Usual and customary debriefers were faculty within their respective campuses, trained in simulation and familiar with debriefing. These debriefers used NLN debriefing questions that were part of the ACE.S teaching resources.

Four students were randomly assigned to roles in every scenario: primary nurse, secondary nurse, and safety sentinel/observer. Following each scenario, students took a small break and then participated in the debriefings. The total time for the simulation lab experience was four hours for the DML intervention group and three hours for the usual and customary control group.

Instruments

Health Sciences Reasoning Test (HSRT)

The first research question asked about the impact of a faculty-facilitated, guided, reflective teaching method to enhance students' development of clinical reasoning skills during a geriatric simulation learning experience. Clinical reasoning was measured using the HSRT (Facione & Facione, 2006), a 33-question, validated, multiple-choice test designed to assess critical-thinking skills in health science students (undergraduate and graduate) and professional health science practitioners. With the HSRT, students draw inferences, make interpretations, analyze information, identify claims and reasons, and evaluate the quality of arguments. Scores are reported for: analysis, inference, evaluation, induction, deduction, and overall reasoning skills, the same critical-thinking subscales as the California Critical Thinking Skills Test (CCTST). The overall reasoning skill score targets the strength or weakness of one's skill in making reflective, reasoned judgments about what to believe or what to do without requiring health care knowledge.

Reliability is established for the HSRT using the Kuder-Richardson 20-calculation for dichotomous multidimensional scales. Overall internal consistency reliability estimates range from .77 to .84 (Facione & Facione, 2006). Content and construct validity were established by correlating test items to the Delphi Report along with support from health sciences faculty committees and human resources professionals as well as national and international graduate research (American Philosophical Association, 1990; Facione & Facione, 2006). At the time of this study, criterion validity statistics for the HSRT were not available (Facione & Facione, 2006).

Debriefing Assessment for Simulation in Healthcare–Student Version (DASH©–SV)

The DASH-SV was used to answer the second research question, on nursing students' perceptions of the quality of debriefing. The DASH–SV (Simon, Raemer, & Rudolph, 2009) was designed to rate six key elements of a debriefing, including whether and how the instructor: (a) establishes an engaging learning environment, (b) maintains an engaging learning environment, (c) structures debriefing in an organized way, (d) provokes engaging discussions, (e) identifies and explores performance gaps, and (f) helps trainees achieve or sustain good future performance. Dreifuerst (2012) reported that initial reliability of the DASH-SV was completed during her original study. She reported findings of 0.82 ($n = 6$, $M = 29.54$, variance $= 24.26$, $SD = 4.93$). Criterion and content validity were established by the developers (Simon et al., 2009).

RESULTS

This study investigated two research questions. The first research question, on whether the DML debriefing method would positively impact the development of clinical reasoning skills in undergraduate nursing students, was tested using data from the HSRT. The findings are as follows: pre-test, intervention group ($n = 78$, $M = 22.74$, $SD = 3.6$) and control group ($n = 75$, $M = 22.06$, $SD = 3.7$); post-test, after the simulation and debriefing, intervention group ($n = 78$, $M = 23.56$, $SD = 3.9$) and control group ($n = 75$, $M = 22.41$, $SD = 4.6$).

The change in the mean score for students in the intervention group analyzed using a simple paired t-test resulted in a p-value of .03 and was determined to be significant at the .05 level. The change in mean scores for the students in the control group analyzed using a simple paired t-test resulted in a p-value of .44 and was determined to be insignificant. The change in mean scores between the intervention and control groups analyzed using a simple paired t-test rendered a p-value of .09 and was determined to be significant at the .10 level. (See Table 9.1.)

Nursing students who had the DML debriefing scored significantly higher in their clinical reasoning than nursing students who had usual and customary debriefing. Controlling for change over time, the difference was examined further using analysis of variance (ANOVA). The improvement in scores shown by the treatment group over and above what these students would have achieved over time without DML was found to be statistically insignificant with a reported p-value of .23.

Reporting on the statistical analysis overall, it is important to note that, when controlling for the pre-test, there is a significant change in scores from pre- to post-test that is not recognized in the control group. Second, while the magnitude in the change is not large and the result is not robust, given a small sample size, even a small change or difference can be interpreted as an important trend.

The second research question asked whether students would perceive a difference in the quality of debriefing when the DML method is used compared to usual and customary debriefing. Quality of debriefing was examined using scores from the DASH-SV: intervention group ($n = 78$, $M = 37.45$, $SD = 3.66$); control group ($n = 75$, $M = 35.95$, $SD = 5.20$). The change in mean scores between the intervention and control groups

TABLE 9.1

HSRT Change in Mean Score

t-Test: Paired Two-Sample for Means	Treatment		Control		Post-Score t-Test: Two-Sample Assuming Equal Variances		
	Pre	Post	Pre	Post		Treatment	Control
Mean	22.74	23.56	22.01	22.41	Mean	23.56	22.41
Variance	12.79	15.11	13.85	21.57	Variance	15.11	21.57
Observations	78	78	75	75	Observations	78	75
					Pooled Variance	18.27	
df	77		74		df	151	
t Stat	−2.25		−0.78		t Stat	−1.66	
P(T <= t) one-tail	0.014		0.22		P(T <= t) one-tail	0.05	
t Critical one-tail	1.66		1.67		t Critical one-tail	1.65	
P(T <= t) two-tail	**0.03**		**0.44**		P(T <= t) two-tail	**0.09**	
t Critical two-tail	1.99		1.99		t Critical two-tail	1.98	

analyzed using a simple paired *t*-test resulted in a *p*-value of .04 and was significant at the .05 level. (See Table 9.2.) Students involved in DML debriefing perceived a positive difference in the quality of the debriefing compared with students who experienced the usual and customary debriefing.

TABLE 9.2

DASH-SV Mean Score Change

DASH-SV
t-Test: Two-Sample Assuming Equal Variances

	Treatment	Control
Mean	37.45	35.95
Variance	13.36	26.99
Observations	78	75
Pooled Variance	20.18	
df	148	
t Stat	2.05	
P(T <= t) one-tail	0.02	
t Critical one-tail	1.65	
P(T <= t) two-tail	**0.04**	
t Critical two-tail	1.98	

DISCUSSION

If a major goal in nursing education is to teach students to think like a nurse, teaching strategies need to role model this thinking—guiding the learner to transfer their learning to the practice setting to ultimately improve patient care outcomes. This can only be accomplished if learners understand how to employ their knowledge to make contextually relevant connections in new situations (Schön, 1983; Tennyson, 1992). In this study, Debriefing for Meaningful Learning had a positive impact on the development of clinical reasoning skills in undergraduate nursing students when compared to usual and customary debriefing. Faculty were able to role model a pattern of thinking and dialogue. The debriefing emphasized how similar stories in different contexts require similar thinking and reasoning—a primary learning principle in assisting students to begin to transfer their learning (Schön, 1983; Tennyson, 1992).

In the landmark nursing simulation study conducted by the National Council of State Boards of Nursing (Hayden, Smiley, Alexander, Kardong-Edgren, & Jeffries, 2014), four important qualifiers were deemed necessary to achieve positive learning outcomes when using simulation and debriefing. These include the use of: International Nursing Association for Clinical Simulation and Learning (INACSL) Standards of Best Practice (INACSL, 2013), high-quality simulations, trained and dedicated simulation faculty, and debriefing methods grounded in educational theory.

Findings from this study illustrate that students perceived DML as a higher quality debriefing experience when compared with usual and customary debriefing. Hayden et al. (2014) contend that high quality simulation and debriefing are required to achieve positive learning outcomes. Similarly, Jeffries (2005) outlines principles for sound education practice in the NLN/Jeffries Simulation Framework to assist educators in developing, implementing, and evaluating simulation. These principles include active learning, feedback, student/faculty interaction, collaboration, high expectations, diverse learning, and time on task. This study was guided by a solid debriefing framework and utilized these principles to provide structure and positively influence student learning outcomes.

Finally, the positive change in clinical reasoning was achieved across multiple settings with multiple facilitators. Groups of students had the opportunity to test the debriefing interventions in familiar surroundings, but with debriefing facilitators with whom they were not familiar. Dreifuerst (2012) explains that a possible difference in scores between the intervention and control groups *in her study* may have been due, in part, to the confounding variable of a single facilitator/debriefer.

The role of the facilitator and debriefer cannot be underestimated in connection with learners' perceptions of effectiveness. If only one debriefer is involved, how does one account for factors such as familiarity? This study utilized a carefully designed multisite implementation plan that: controlled for familiarity of the debriefer across settings and trained for and implemented a consistent method of debriefing. Consequently, the positive effect seen across multiple sites was the result of the DML method rather than the effect of a single debriefer.

Limitations

This study was intended to replicate Dreifuerst's (2012) findings of a positive change in clinical reasoning using the DML methodology. The HSRT assesses health professionals and not nursing specifically. Therefore, it may not adequately assess the nature of the clinical reasoning used by nurses in practice. The findings of the study are limited because the total number of subjects fell below the anticipated sample size needed to enhance power. A larger sample size would have increased the strength and generalizability of the findings.

Implications for Nursing Education

Oermann et al. (2012) discuss the importance of multisite studies. While multiple settings improve the generalizability of the findings, managing consistency and rigor is challenging and requires a thoughtful and meticulous approach. This study had very specific implementation and training procedures that were successfully executed across four geographically separated nursing programs. The use of standardized simulation scenarios, debriefing methods, and evaluation measures greatly contributed to this study's consistency and rigor. High-quality simulation and debriefing requires utilization of piloted, tested, and standardized resources. This is an important consideration for both nursing education and research.

The literature contains only a few single-site studies employing the use of DML. These studies suggest that further research across different settings and with larger populations are needed to inform our understanding of debriefing on nursing student learning and behavior (Dreifuerst, 2009, 2012; Mariani et al., 2013). This multisite study adds to the understanding and impact of theory-based debriefing on clinical reasoning. Further research across multiple settings with larger populations is warranted.

Finally, Debriefing for Meaningful Learning as an effective debriefing method highlights the importance of reflection and our roles as educators in guiding students and role modeling "thinking like a nurse." The findings of this study produced simulation evaluation evidence at the level of impacting student learning, that is, Kirkpatrick's Level 2 (1994). Further research is needed to capture the transfer of learning to the clinical setting and ultimately, how the DML directly improves patient care outcomes (Adamson et al., 2013).

CONCLUSION

The study reported here involved a theory-based method of debriefing that was implemented across multiple sites. The use of high-quality simulation and debriefing methods IS necessary if we are going to enhance student learning and, ultimately, clinical reasoning. Trained faculty guided students through a debriefing experience that engaged a critical conversation—making known the rationale behind thinking—a type of conversation that is essential in nursing education today. It is hoped that the findings of this multisite study will continue to advance the dialogue in nursing education on meaningful learning and the development of clinical reasoning in nursing students.

References

Adamson, K. A., Kardong-Edgren, S., & Willhaus, J. (2013). An updated review of published simulation evaluation instruments. *Clinical Simulation in Nursing, 9*(9), e393–e400. doi:0.1016/j.ecns.2012.09.004

American Philosophical Association, Committee on Pre-College Philosophy. (1990). *Critical thinking: A statement of expert consensus for purposes of educational assessment and instruction: The Delphi report.* New York, NY: Author.

Bybee, R. W., Buchwald, C. E., Crissman, S., Heil, D. R., Kuebis, P. J., Matsumoto, C., & McInerney, J. D. (1989). *Science and technology education for the elementary years: Frameworks for curriculum and instruction.* Washington, DC: National Center for Improving Science Education.

Cantrell, M. A. (2008). The importance of debriefing in clinical simulations. *Clinical Simulation in Nursing, 4*(2), e19–e23. doi:10.1016/j.ecns.2008.06.006

Cicero, M. X., Auerbach, M. A., Zigmont, J., Riera, A., Ching, K., & Baum, C. R. (2012). Simulation training with structured debriefing improves residents' pediatric disaster triage performance. *Prehospital Disaster Medicine, 27*(3), 239–244.

Decker, S. (2007). Integrating guided reflection into simulated learning experiences. In P. R. Jeffries (Ed.), *Simulation in Nursing* (pp. 73–85). New York, NY: The National League for Nursing.

Dreifuerst, K. T. (2009). The essentials of debriefing in simulation learning: A concept analysis. *Nursing Education Perspectives, 30*(2), 109–114.

Dreifuerst, K. T. (2012). Using debriefing for meaningful learning to foster development of clinical reasoning in simulation. *Journal of Nursing Education, 51*(6), 326–333.

Facione, N. C., & Facione, P. A. (2006). *The health sciences reasoning test (HSRT): A test of critical thinking skills for health care professionals.* Millbrae, CA: California Academic Press.

Fanning, R. M., & Gaba, D. M. (2007). The role of debriefing in simulation-based learning. *Simulation in Healthcare, 2*(2), 115–125.

Faul, F., Erdfelder, E., Buchner, A., & Lang, A. G. (2009). Statistical power analyses using G*Power 3.1: Tests for correlation and regression analyses. *Behavior Research Methods, 41*, 1149–1160.

Forneris, S. G. (2004). Exploring the attributes of critical thinking: A conceptual basis. *International Journal of Nursing Education Scholarship. 1*(1, Article 9), 1–18.

Forneris, S. G., & Peden-McAlpine, C. (2006) Contextual learning: A reflective learning intervention for nursing education. *International Journal of Nursing Education Scholarship 3*(1, article 17), 1–18.

Forneris, S. G., & Peden-McAlpine, C. (2007). Evaluation of a reflective learning intervention to improve critical thinking in novice nurses. *Journal of Advanced Nursing 57*(4), 1–12.

Hayden, J. K., Smiley, R. A., Alexander, M., Kardong-Edgren, S., & Jeffries, P. R. (2014). The NCSBN national simulation study: A longitudinal, randomized, controlled study replacing clinical hours with simulation in prelicensure nursing education. *Journal of Nursing Regulation, 5*(2), Suppl, S3–S40.

International Nursing Association for Clinical Simulation and Learning (INACSL). (2013). Standards of Best Practice: Simulation. *Clinical Simulation in Nursing, 9*(6), Suppl, Sii–Siii.

Jeffries, P. R. (2005). A framework for designing, implementing, and evaluating simulations used as teaching strategies in nursing. *Nursing Education Perspectives, 26*(2), 96–103. doi:10.1043/1536-5026(2005)026<0096:AFWFDI>2.0.CO;2

Jeffries, P. R. (Ed.). (2012). *Simulation in nursing education: From conceptualization to evaluation* (2nd ed.). New York, NY: the National League for Nursing.

Kirkpatrick, D. L. (1994). *Evaluating training programs: The four levels.* San Francisco, CA: Bernett-Koehler.

Kolb, D. A. (1984). *Experiential learning: Experience as the source of learning and development.* Englewood Clifts, NJ: Prentice-Hall.

Kuiper, R., Heinrich, C., Matthias, A., Graham, M. J., & Bell-Kotwell, L. (2008). Debriefing with the OPT model of clinical reasoning during high fidelity patient simulation. *International Journal of Nursing Education Scholarship, 5*(1), Article 17. doi:10.2202/1548-923X.1466

Lasater, K. (2007) Clinical judgment development: Using simulation to create an assessment rubric. *Journal of Nursing Education, 46*(11), 496–503.

Lipsey, M. W. (1990). *Design sensitivity: Statistical power for experimental research.* Newbury Park, CA: Sage.

Mariani, B., Cantrell, M. A., Meakim, C., Prieto, P., & Dreifuerst, K. T. (2013). Structured debriefing and students' clinical judgment abilities in simulation. *Clinical Simulation in Nursing, 9*(5), e147–e155. doi:10.1016/j.ecns.2011.11.009

Myrick, F., & Yonge, O. (2002). Preceptor questioning and student critical thinking. *Journal of Professional Nursing, 18*(3), 176–181.

Myrick, F., & Yonge, O. (2003). Enhancing critical thinking in the preceptorship experience in nursing education. *Journal of Advanced Nursing 45*(4), 371–380.

The National League for Nursing. (2012). *NLN Research Priorities in Nursing Education 2012–2015.* Retrieved from www.nln.org/docs/default-source/default-document-library/researchpriorities.pdf?sfvrsn=2

Neill, M. A., & Wotton, K. (2011). High-fidelity simulation debriefing in nursing education: A literature review. *Clinical Simulation in Nursing, 7*, e161–e168. doi:10.1016/j.ecns.2011.02.001

Oermann, M. H., Hallmark, B. F., Haus, C., Kardong-Edgren, S. E., Keegan McColgan, J., & Rogers, N. (2012). Conducting multisite research studies in nursing education: Brief practice of CPR skills as an exemplar. *Journal of Nursing Education, 51*(1), 23–28.

Parker, B., & Myrick, F. (2010). Transformative learning as a context for human patient simulation. *Journal of Nursing Education, 49*(6), 326–332.

Reese, C. R. (2010). *ACES Case #1: Millie Larsen* (developed by the National League for Nursing, Simulation Team Advancing Gerontological Education Strategies [STAGES]). Retrieved from www.nln.org/professional-development-programs/teaching-resources/aging/ace-s/unfolding-cases/millie-larsen

Schön, D. A. (1983). *The reflective practitioner: How professionals think in action.* New York, NY: Basic Books.

Schön, D. A. (1987). *Educating the reflective practitioner.* San Francisco, CA: Jossey-Bass.

Shinnick, M. A., Woo, M., Horwich, T. B., & Steadman, R. (2011). Debriefing: The most important component in simulation? *Clinical Simulation in Nursing, 7*(3), e105–e111. doi:10.1016/j.ecns.2010.11.005

Simon, R., Raemer D. B., & Rudolph, J. W. (2009). *Debriefing assessment for simulation in healthcare.* Boston, MA: Center for Medical Simulation.

Tanner, C. (2006). Thinking like a nurse: A research-based model of clinical judgment in nursing. *Journal of Nursing Education, 45*(6), 204–211.

Tennyson, R. D. (1992). An educational learning theory for instructional design. *Educational Technology, 32*(1), 36–41.

10

Clinical Application of ACE.S and the ACE.S Design Tree

Michele Cislo, MA, RN

The NLN Advancing Care Excellence for Seniors (ACE.S) program has provided the students of Union County College Practical Nursing Department with an "ah-ha" moment. Use of this program within the Practical Nursing program has provided our students with a more organized approach to patient care. The Design Tree was developed in conjunction with the ACE.S teaching resources and has taken the implementation to a higher level, with students having a greater ability to organize and prioritize patient care.

STRUCTURE OF PROGRAM

Before beginning to utilize the ACE.S unfolding cases, students in the first nursing class listen to Maria Diaz's monologue; Maria discusses her experience with multiple chronic health problems consistent with geriatric syndromes. This activity is coordinated with a class on communication skills. As a group project, students discuss Maria's monologue, generating a Geriatric Syndromes concept map on a classroom whiteboard. Students are then assigned to conduct an interview with an older adult, using the guide that is available on the ACE.S website, under Teaching Strategies (Caring for the Older Adult in the Community). Students discuss their interviews in class; it is interesting to note that, after listening to Maria's monologue, they more readily identify geriatric syndromes. Besides enjoying the experience, students have found out more things about their older relatives and acquaintances, sharing comments such as, "I hadn't realized that my grandfather enjoys going to the food store. From now on, rather than just getting a shopping list, I am going to take him to the store every couple of weeks from now on."

Integration of ACE.S and the unfolding case studies has led to students' developing a more comprehensive skill set and accomplishing course learning outcomes more readily. Faculty attribute this to the personalization of the learning process with more realistic patient scenarios. The students' approach to patient care is more holistic, rather than focusing on the medical model.

"Red" Yoder is one of the case studies that faculty have chosen to utilize for the entire practical nursing program. "Red" was chosen because, as the simulation scenarios increase in complexity, students also are able to advance and more readily assimilate skills that transfer to the clinical setting. The first "Red" Yoder simulation is utilized in the fundamentals course, with the students working in groups and analyzing data based on the debriefing guide from the Instructor's Toolkit. Students continue to participate in the subsequent "Red" Yoder simulation modules in the next semesters. In addition to group discussions, students practice skills such as insulin injection and wound care using practice "Red" mannequins. The How to Try This videos are used throughout the curriculum to coincide with the appropriate classroom topics, such as patient safety.

DEVELOPMENT OF THE DESIGN TREE CONCEPT MAP

Faculty recognized that there was a need to facilitate the transition of learning from the simulation lab to the clinical setting. The ACE.S Design Tree was created to assist students to gain a more holistic picture of patient care and to utilize alternative assessment tools more effectively. For example, prior to its introduction, clinical assignments focused on the patient's acute problem. For example, the clinical instructor may have assigned a patient with a fractured ankle, with the student concentrating much of the time on the orthopedic nature of this health alteration. After instituting ACE.S and using the ACE.S Design Tree, students have expanded their plan of care by including the impact of the underlying comorbidities, the patient's vulnerabilities during transitions, and the individuality of each patient. Faculty also noticed that, before instituting use of the ACE.S Design Tree, students would often administer the SPICES© tool, for example, and obtain the data, but then verbalize confusion regarding what to do next or how the patient's individual situation would factor into the nursing plan of care. Using the ACE.S Design Tree concept map helped students to recognize that an older adult may have an acute illness with multiple underlying chronic health problems (Figure 10.1).

COMPONENTS OF THE ACE.S DESIGN TREE CONCEPT MAP
Patient Data

Post-conference discussions focused on the four categories of patient data that appear in the Design Tree concept map. The first category is the identification of the acute episode or what brought this patient into the health care setting. Indicating the patient's primary medical concern is certainly not a new practice, but the ACE.S program helped us to understand the importance of focusing on more than the acute care episode to foster individualized care for older adults. The next three categories in the Design Tree concept map—chronic illness, caregiver responsibilities, and medications—help students to recognize the individuality of each patient. Students identify appropriate data in each of these three boxes.

Tools
SPICES© Tool

Next, the SPICES© Tool is used by students for further patient assessment. Student feedback regarding the use of the SPICES© tool was positive; however, faculty noticed

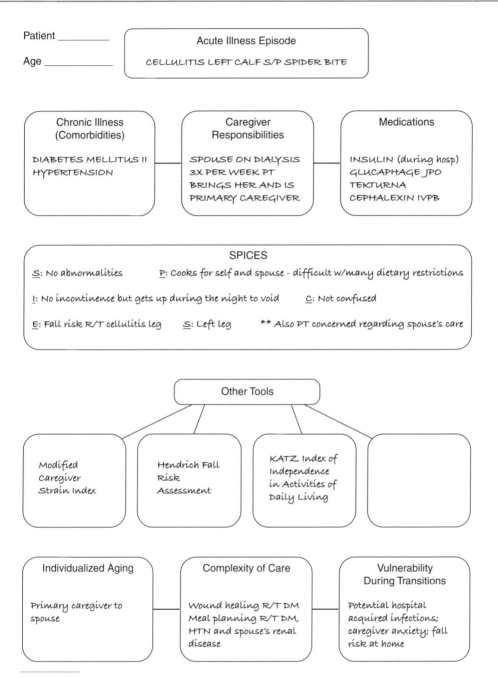

Patient _____

Age _____

Acute Illness Episode

CELLULITIS LEFT CALF S/P SPIDER BITE

Chronic Illness (Comorbidities)

DIABETES MELLITUS II
HYPERTENSION

Caregiver Responsibilities

SPOUSE ON DIALYSIS
3X PER WEEK PT
BRINGS HER AND IS
PRIMARY CAREGIVER

Medications

INSULIN (during hosp)
GLUCAPHAGE JPO
TEKTURNA
CEPHALEXIN IVPB

SPICES

S: No abnormalities   P: Cooks for self and spouse - difficult w/many dietary restrictions

I: No incontinence but gets up during the night to void   C: Not confused

E: Fall risk R/T cellulitis leg   S: Left leg   ** Also PT concerned regarding spouse's care

Other Tools

Modified
Caregiver
Strain Index

Hendrich Fall
Risk
Assessment

KATZ Index of
Independence
in Activities of
Daily Living

Individualized Aging

Primary caregiver to
spouse

Complexity of Care

Wound healing R/T DM
Meal planning R/T DM,
HTN and spouse's renal
disease

Vulnerability During Transitions

Potential hospital
acquired infections;
caregiver anxiety; fall
risk at home

FIGURE 10.1 The ACE.S Design Tree concept map. (Copyright © 2014 Michele Cislo, UCC Practical Nursing Department.)

a disconnect between interpreting data collected from the SPICES© tool and the next step of assessment.

Other Tools

The students verbalized confusion regarding which tool(s) should be utilized next to obtain more complete patient information. To facilitate more accurate assessment and promote effective care, a listing of tools by category, was added on the reverse side of the Design Tree tool (Box 10.1). This allows students to choose the next assessment tool

---

BOX 10.1

ACE.S Further Assessment Tools (See also ConsultGeriRN.org)

After completing SPICES tool, choose any of the following appropriate tools for further assessment.

ADLs
Katz index for Independent Living

Dementia
Pain Assessment in People with Dementia
Pain Assessment in Older Adults

Hospital Admission
Hospital Admission Risk Profile
Reducing Functional Decline in Older Adults

Immunizations for the Older Adult

Psychosocial Tools
Mini-Cog
Montreal Cognitive Assessment
Geriatric Depression Scale
Detecting Delirium-CAM
The Impact of Event Scale
Horowitz Impact of Event Sale

Skin
Braden Scale-Predicting Pressure Ulcer Risk

Sleep
Assessment of Fatigue in Older Adults
Pittsburg Sleep Quality Index
Epsworth Sleep Scale

Pain
Assessing Pain in Older Adults

Fall Risk
Hendrich Fall Risk Assessment
Assessment of Fear of Falling

Sexuality
Sexuality Assessment For Older Adults

Alcohol Abuse
Alcohol Use and Screening Assessment
Alcohol Use & Misuse in Older Adults

Urinary Incontinence
Transient Urinary Incontinence in the Older
    Adult
Persistent Urinary Incontinence

Hearing Screening
Hearing Screening in Older Adults
A Brief Hearing Loss Screen

Caregivers
Modified Caregiver Strain Index

Elder Mistreatment
Elder Mistreatment Assessment

Spirituality
Related Resources from the Hospice and
Palliative Nurses Association

Oral Health/ Dysphagia

Kayser-Jones Brief Oral Status Exam
Preventing Aspiration in Older Adults with
    Dysphagia

Beers Criteria for Potentially Inappropriate Medications Used for Older Adults

to administer to the patient, based upon their presenting health issues. For example, prior to using the Design Tree and ACE.S tools, for a patient with a fall risk the student would obtain a yellow wristband and place a yellow star outside the patient's room, according to policy at the health care facility. Using the tools takes the assessment one step further, with the risk of falls being followed through to the discharge plan.

Plan of Care

After administering the selected tools and completing the information in the Design Tree, students generate a plan of care. The NLN Essential Knowledge Domains are utilized to formulate patient outcomes. Students identify individualized aging and what is unique about the particular patient, such as caring for an ill spouse. The second category, complexity of care, reflects other factors that will influence the patient's ongoing recovery. Vulnerability during transitions identifies potential areas of concern, such as susceptibility to infection and risk of falls. The patient's vulnerability will always include review and acknowledgment of the National Patient Safety Goals (The Joint Commission, 2016). This piece stimulates much discussion and student learning, as many patient concerns are highlighted and included in the planning for care in the health care agency and at home.

The Design Tree mirrors the current trend in healthcare communication based on Atul Gawande's Checklist Manifesto (2009), such as the bundle checklists for procedures and the "Time Out" protocols which stress the importance of outlining steps to follow to ensure comprehensive patient care. The Design Tree and the ACE.S teaching resources stimulate the student, and then the graduate nurse, to realign priorities as the individual situation necessitates for the patient's optimal health. The role of the LPN will be predominant in caring for the "silver tsunami" (Tagliareni, et al., 2012) as the aging population increases in numbers. Ultimately, it is our hope that use of the ACE.S program and Design Tree will change our graduate's ability to more fully assess and intervene for a healthier older adult population. An email from a graduate practicing with the elder population writes, "I use all the skills I learned. But the ACE.S Design Tree and the tools from the ACE.S and ConsultGeri websites really showed me how to assess the older adult completely. I am sharing this knowledge with my co-workers, as the success of my care is evident."

References

ConsultGeri. (2016). *Try This Series.* Retrieved from www.consultgeri.org

Gawande, Atul. (2009). *The Checklist Manifesto,* New York, NY: Picador Publishing.

The Joint Commission. (2016). National Patient Safety Goals.Retrieved from http://www.jointcommission.org/assets/1/6/2016_NPSG_HAP_ER.pdf

Quality Safety and Education for Nurses. (2016). Prelicensure KSA's (Knowledge, Skills and Attitudes). Retrieved from www.qsen.org

Tagliareni, E., King, E., Mengel, A., & McLaughlin, B. (2012). Quality care for older adults. The NLN Advancing Care Excellence for Seniors (ACE.S) Project. *Nursing Education Perspectives, 33*(3) 144–149.

11

ACE.S Unfolding Case Simulations Redesigned to Address Family Nursing Care Competencies for Older Adults

Norma Krumwiede, EdD, MEd, MN, RN

Colleen Royle, EdD, MSN, RN

Kelly Krumwiede, PhD, RN, PHN

Stacey Van Gelderen, DNP, RN

MaryAnn McKenna Moon, MSN, APRN, ACNS-BC

Walter Groteluschen, MS

OVERVIEW

Recent developments in family nursing offer direction to nurse educators in refining simulation learning to more fully engage students in developing confidence and competence in a nursing practice focused on families. This chapter will identify how one academic system guides students' simulation learning experiences through unfolding cases that integrate family experiences and processes in order to achieve family nursing competencies that ensure quality nursing care with families.

DEVELOPMENT AND IMPLEMENTATION

Research findings highlight the significance of the family to the health and well-being of individual aging members, as well as the influence of a senior member's illness on the family (Price, Bush, & Price, 2017; Chesla, 2010). Despite increasing knowledge of the importance of family nursing, research continues to report deficiencies in the current state of family nursing practice (Duhamel, 2010; Svavarsdottir et al., 2015). It is possible that gaps in senior care are rooted in a lack of formal education about family-focused nursing in contemporary curricula. Nursing education has yet to fully develop approaches and strategies for teaching family nursing practice in simulation teaching and learning experiences (Eggenberger, Krumwiede, & Young, 2015a). Simulation pedagogy in many academic and practice systems primarily focuses on technical skills, rather than family nursing or relational skills (Eggenberger & Regan, 2010). Yet, simulation learning experiences offer prime opportunities to advance nursing practice with families.

The International Family Nursing Association (IFNA) published position statements on Pre-licensure Family Nursing Education (IFNA, 2013) and Generalist Competencies for Family Nursing Practice (IFNA, 2015) that encourage nurse educators to include family throughout pre-licensure nursing education. These statements offer direction for refining simulation learning to more fully engage students in developing confidence and competence in a nursing practice focused on families. This chapter describes how one faculty team integrated the IFNA position statements with the NLN ACE.S Essential Knowledge Domains and Essential Nursing Actions, using the ACE.S Unfolding Cases, in order to maximize the full potential of learning during these simulations.

Simulation pedagogy offers an innovative opportunity for nurse educators to guide students in developing knowledge of family health and illness experiences and applying family nursing practice and nurse-family interaction skills in real life practice. Nurse educators who want to plan simulation learning experiences to teach family-focused nursing care of older adults can begin by asking questions such as:

1. What do students need to understand about family, family experiences, and family practice in relation to individualized aging?

2. In what ways can my interactions with students instruct and model family-focused care, assist students to think family throughout their learning experience, and use an ecological perspective to understand the complexities of older adults?

3. How can this simulated experience be used to assist students to reflect about their personal actions and identify how factors such as values, judgment, and assumptions can become barriers to providing family-focused care to the older adult population?

Simulation learning in this curriculum includes carefully designed scenarios that incorporate family-focused nursing actions with health and illness situations that undergraduate nursing students often encounter. Students are guided to *Think Family* throughout the older adult simulation learning experiences which support their achievement of family nursing competencies, for example, ensuring the quality of nursing care with families in everyday practices (Denham, Eggenberger, Young, & Krumwiede, 2015). Faculty coach students to develop confidence in establishing nurse-family relationship skills and provide competent and caring nursing actions focused on the family as the recipient of care. This perspective helps students to value the family as supportive to the family member with an illness and understand the concerns of the family when a family member has an illness (Eggenberger et al., 2015).

Scenarios refined by faculty address Family Nursing Care Competencies for older adults include developing a nursing practice focused on: (a) Family strengths and mobilizing family resources, (b) Family self-management and facilitating life transitions, (c) Committing to a self-reflective practice based on examination of the nurse actions with families and family responses, and (d) an evidence-based approach. Students practice nursing actions (Wright & Leahey, 2013) during scenarios that focus on competencies, such as:

> Engaging and including family members in therapeutic conversations and care;

> Utilizing therapeutic communication techniques with families;

> Incorporating useful questions in their nursing practice with families;

> Performing family assessments that include health issues, family beliefs, family dynamics, and family strengths; and

> Incorporating health promotion and illness management with family members and the family unit.

Each simulation scenario includes several strategies to prepare the student for their learning experience. A prerecorded audio monologue is used to introduce the older adult patient and their family members to the students. A learning packet consisting of pertinent evidence-based articles or text readings that address family nursing research is provided. This School of Nursing developed a Family Nursing Constructs Framework (Eggenberger, Krumwiede, & Young, 2015a; Eggenberger, Krumwiede, & Meiers, 2015b) to guide faculty in using family nursing evidence and encourage undergraduate nursing students to care for families and improve the health of society. The Family Nursing Constructs Framework was created as a coherent approach to guide teaching family-focused nursing actions in our curriculum. Constructs that address family illness experiences and related family-focused nursing actions are provided electronically within the learning management system prior to the simulation experience.

Students acting as family members during simulations are given cue cards with prompts to guide the students to learning outcomes related to family experiences during illness. Box 11.1 contains a family cue card for Red Yoder's daughter-in-law, Judy, prompting the students to foster a further assessment regarding Red's sleep patterns, alcohol use, diet, and medication. These cues should prompt the nursing student to use the Hartford tools: SPICES, Pittsburgh Sleep Quality Index, Katz Index of Independence in Activities of Daily Living, and Alcohol Use and Screening Tool (How to Try This Series, 2016).

Students are also encouraged to use family measures that examine particular aspects of family processes, and functioning or health from the family member or

BOX 11.1

Family Cue Card for Red Yoder's Daughter-in-Law, Judy

Red Yoder Scenario 1

Scenario #1 Judy, Daughter-in-Law

5–10 min: Judy is supportive and brings up issues to guide the assessment.
Did you say you have trouble sleeping?
When I got your groceries, you wanted more beer than you usually drink in a week.
You take a few other medications don't you?
Did you have bacon and eggs again for breakfast today?

BOX 11.2

Family Awareness and Sensitivity Tool

1. When did you feel most cared for or cared about in this scenario?
2. When did you feel least cared for or cared about?
3. How did playing the role of a family member increase your understanding of the family's illness experience?
4. Which nursing actions did you experience during the scenario that you want to incorporate into your family-focused practice?
5. What actions did the nurse take that made you feel included and comforted? What actions were not helpful?

---

family unit perspective. These measures and tools, such as Family Hardiness or Family Assessment Devices may address specific family constructs such as resilience and communication or overall family functioning and health (Sawin & Harrigan, 1995). Other scales that explore the experience of a family with chronic illness, such as The Family Illness Experience Scale: Chronic Illness (Meiers, Eggenberger, & Krumwiede, 2016) help students develop directions for care focused on family processes during a chronic illness.

To elicit their emotional responses, faculty encourage students who are role playing a family member to consider past experiences. Family members choose wigs, jewelry, clothing, and other props to provide a realistic environment of care. A verbal report is read by a student portraying the nurse finishing her shift and handing off care with a full SBAR report that includes a family focus component of care. For example, in one case the family's anxiety with the hospitalization of a family member is evident, and the nurse needs to address the family anxiety by listening and explaining the next steps. In the ACE.S Unfolding Case of Millie Larsen, the uncertainty of the family is evident, and the nurse works to identify the strengths and resources of the family to support the transition to home.

As part of the simulation learning experience, students engage in a debriefing reflection time that has a focus on the older adult and their family, family constructs, and family-focused nursing actions. Individualized debriefing tools are created for each scenario to establish a clear path to learning outcomes and family nursing competencies for faculty and students. The Family Awareness and Sensitivity Tool (Krumwiede, Royle, & Moon, 2015; see Box 11.2) assists students who role play family members to share their feelings as a family member which helps students gain understandings of the family experience and actions needed by the nurse to alleviate family distress, manage their role as a protector, or serve as a resource. Particular ACE.S cases are strategically placed throughout the curriculum to enact care of families with an older adult. First-semester juniors experience Millie Larsen and Red Yoder while first-semester seniors experience Henry Williams, and Julia Morales and Lucy Grey.

EVALUATION

An assessment and evaluation process was implemented to analyze the effectiveness of simulation pedagogy, substantiate the replacement of clinical hours with simulation, and explore the impact of the ACE.S unfolding cases on teaching family-focused nursing care of seniors. The quantitative measures consisted of the Knowledge Acquisition Questionnaire (Krumwiede, Royle, & Groteluschen, 2011; see Box 11.4) to assess and evaluate learning during the simulation and the Self-Efficacy Questionnaire (Krumwiede & Royle, 2011; see Box 11.3) modeled after Ravert's dissertation project instrument (pre-/post-survey) that is mapped specifically to each ACE.S case and includes student satisfaction questions. The difference between the means of students' pre- and post-Self-Efficacy Questionnaire responses indicates some statistically significant findings as they relate to the student's knowledge, skills, and abilities regarding several nursing actions. For the 21 self-efficacy items, the average score increased from 55.91 to 65.00. For the 21 knowledge items, the average number correct increased from 13.28 to 17.45. Both were a statistically significant improvement ($p < 0.001$).

BOX 11.3

Self-Efficacy for Millie Larsen: Pre-Questionnaire

DIRECTIONS: Nurses perform many different nursing actions throughout their practice. This survey is measuring your level of confidence to perform various nursing actions. Record your **first reaction:** do not spend a lot of time thinking about each item, rather tell us how confident you are at being able to complete the specific nursing action.

Please check the appropriate column indicating your level of confidence to perform each nursing action.	5 = Extremely Confident	4 = Very Confident	3 = Moderately Confident	2 = Slightly Confident	1 = Not At All Confident
1. Participating in simulated learning experiences					
2. Assessing fall risk (Heindrich II Fall Risk)					
3. Completing symptom assessment: Pain					
4. Communicating with family members					
5. Communicating using the ISBAR technique					
6. Assessing geriatric patient care needs (SPICES)					
7. Assessing IADLs (Katz Index of Independence)					

(continued)

BOX 11.3

Self-Efficacy for Millie Larsen: Pre-Questionnaire (*Continued*)

Please check the appropriate column indicating your level of confidence to perform each nursing action.	5 = Extremely Confident	4 = Very Confident	3 = Moderately Confident	2 = Slightly Confident	1 = Not At All Confident
8. Managing safe medication administration					
9. Monitoring medication use in older adults					
10. Engaging in patient reorientation techniques					
11. Assessing patient's confusion (CAM Confusion Assessment Method)					
12. Identify critical assessment findings					
13. Understanding of lab values for geriatric patients					
14. Assessing for changes in cognition					
15. Completing effective teaching with patient					
16. Completing effective teaching with family					
17. Reviewing a medication reconciliation form					
18. Recognizing common geriatric syndromes (confusion, incontinence, osteoarthritis)					
19. Reviewing the plan of care with patient					
20. Reviewing the plan of care with family					
21. Utilizing evidence based tools to guide your assessment					

BOX 11.3

Self-Efficacy for Millie Larsen: Pre-Questionnaire (*Continued*)

22. How useful was the Millie Larsen simulation packet?	Not useful 1	2	3	4	Very useful 5

23. How many minutes did you spend preparing for today's simulation? _____

24. How confident are you to participate in today's simulation?	Not confident 1	2	3	4	Very confident 5
25. How confident are you to care for a patient with confusion?	Not confident 1	2	3	4	Very confident 5
26. How confident are you to call primary provider for orders?	Not confident 1	2	3	4	Very confident 5
27. How confident are you to communicate with family?	Not confident 1	2	3	4	Very confident 5

Comments:

*Evaluation tool adapted from P. Ravert (2004) dissertation project: Use of a human patient simulator with undergraduate nursing students: A prototype evaluation of critical thinking and self-efficacy.

Faculty have been collecting data that show the impact of educational practices aimed at transforming beliefs and attitudes from the traditional individual focus to a practice that focuses on the family (Young, Krumwiede, & Eggenberger, 2016). A mixed-methods study using a modified Q-methodology design examined attitudes of 15 baccalaureate students graduating from this curriculum. The data analysis revealed four significant factors which represent distinct perspectives including emerging, contesting, engaging, and envisioning family care patterns.

This faculty evaluation of student learning suggests simulation focused on family nursing can advance family nursing practice. Now is the time to embed family nursing skills into simulation design because many nursing programs are designing and evaluating their simulation outcomes. When faculty incorporate the ACE.S Unfolding Case Simulations into their courses, students are more prepared to provide family-focused care. These simulation experiences guide students to gain competencies in family nursing practice that will enhance student learning and have potential to transform nursing practice and foster quality nursing care for older adults and their families.

BOX 11.4

Millie Larsen: Knowledge Acquisition Questionnaire

1. The acronym SPICES refers to six common geriatric syndromes that require nursing interventions. List the six common geriatric syndromes.

   S _____

   P _____

   I _____

   C _____

   E _____

   S _____

2. Nursing staff are trying to provide for the safety of an elderly female client with moderate dementia. She is wandering at night and has trouble keeping her balance. She has fallen twice but has had no resulting injuries. Which intervention is most appropriate?
   a. Move the client to a room near the nurse's station and install a bed alarm.
   b. Have the client sleep in a reclining chair across from the nurse's station.
   c. Help the client to bed and raise all four bedrails.
   d. Ask a family member to stay with the client at night.

3. While educating the daughter of a client with dementia about the illness, the daughter complains to the nurse that her mother distorts things. The nurse understands that the daughter needs further teaching about dementia when she makes which statement?
   a. "I tell her reality, such as, 'That noise is the wind in the trees.'"
   b. "I understand the misperceptions are part of the disease."
   c. "I turn off the radio when we're in another room."
   d. "I tell her she is wrong and then I tell her what's right."

4. Mrs. P is a 76 y.o. diabetic and after a stroke has been relocated to a nursing facility. She has essentially no exercise, is experiencing frequent UTIs, polypharmacy, is a diabetic with a foot ulcer and is under a considerable amount of stress related to her future. During her assessment you found she has urgency related to her UTI. While utilizing the SPICES tool, what part of the case study would be recorded? _____

5. Suzie, an 80 y.o. woman with new onset confusion, anxiety, and UTIs with repeated falls at home over the past two months is hospitalized for observation in consideration of long-term care placement. Upon admission she is anxious, confused and unable to move. She is currently taking Haldol and Ativan BID which were both started one week ago. Her admission lab work was all normal with exception of elevated WBCs and bacteria in her urine. Suzie's Hendrich II score would be:
   a. 9
   b. 6
   c. 7
   d. 8

6. When assessing the Get Up and Go Test, you are aware that it is important to instruct the patient to:
   a. Sit on a chair; have their hands sitting in their lap and ask the patient to stand.
   b. Rise from a lying position; sit at the edge of the bed and then stand.
   c. Begin from the side of the bed and utilize an assistive device to rise to a standing position.
   d. Sit in the chair and rise up while pushing off the arm rest.

BOX 11.4

Millie Larsen: Knowledge Acquisition Questionnaire (*Continued*)

7. When you communicate with the physician to inform her that Millie has become confused, you utilize ISBARR. The acronym ISBARR refers to:

    I _____

    S _____

    B _____

    A _____

    R _____

    R _____

8. Kathy is a 56 year old lady who was admitted yesterday to a general ward of a small rural hospital. She was admitted for investigation of increasing shortness of breath after a recent URTI. Her past medical history includes morbid obesity (weight = 124 kg), Type 2 diabetes, hypertension (normal blood pressure 150/85 mmHg), and asthma. Her medications include anti-hypertensives, a cholesterol-lowering agent and oral hypoglycemics. Kathy also uses a bronchodilator puffer as required. She has been using her puffer more often. Kathy has a complex social history, and presents to the Emergency Department several times per year. On admission, her observations were: respiratory rate 18; Oxygen saturation by pulse oximetry (SpO2) 96%; blood pressure 146/80; heart rate 96. As a nurse comfortable in using the ISBARR reporting format you understand that her conditions of diabetes, morbid obesity, hypertension, and asthma are from which part of the ISBARR reporting tool?

    a. _____

9. The Katz instrument can be effectively used among older adults in a variety of care settings to assess:

    a. Confusion, dressing, toileting, transferring, continence, and feeding

    b. Gait, dressing, toileting, transferring, continence, and feeding

    c. Bathing, dressing, toileting, transferring, continence, and feeding

    d. Medications, disease processes, level of independence, social resources, and financial stability

10. Suzie, an 80 y.o. woman with new onset confusion, anxiety, and UTIs with repeated falls at home over the past two months is hospitalized for observation in consideration of long-term care placement. Upon admission she is anxious, confused and unable to move. She is currently taking Haldol and Ativan BID which were both started one week ago. Her admission lab work was all normal with exception of elevated WBCs and bacteria in her urine. Suzie has made outstanding progress during her hospitalization you are preparing to discharge her to home and you desire to assess her ability to provide self-care on a daily basis. Which of the following tools would be most helpful in assessing these abilities:

    a. Hendrich II

    b. KATZ

    c. CAM

    d. Elder Mistreatment Assessment

References

Chesla, C. (2010). Do family interventions improve health? *Journal of Family Nursing, 16*(4), 355–377. doi: 10.1177/1074840710383145

Denham, S. A., Eggenberger, S. K., Young, P. K., & Krumwiede, N. K. (Eds.). (2016). *Family-focused care: Think family and transform nursing practice*. Philadelphia: F. A. Davis.

Duhamel, F. (2010). Implementing family nursing: How do we translate knowledge into clinical practice? Part II: The evolution of 20 years of teaching, research, and practice to a Center of Excellence in Family Nursing. *Journal of Family Nursing, 16*(1), 8–25.

Eggenberger, S. K., Krumwiede, N. K., &Young, P. K. (2015a). Using simulation pedagogy in the formation of family-focused generalist nurses. *Journal of Nursing Education, 54*(10), 588–593.

Eggenberger, S. K., Krumwiede, N. K., & Meiers, S. J. (2015b, August). Family nursing construct framework links research, education and practice. Paper presentation at the 12th International Family Nursing Conference, Odense, Denmark.

Eggenberger, S. K., & Regan, M. (2010). Expanding simulation to teach family nursing. *Journal of Nursing Education, 49*(10), 550–558.

How to Try This Series. (2016). Lippincott Learning Center. Retrieved from http://www.nursingcenter. com/static?pageid=730390&utm_ source=WhatCountsEmail&utm_ medium=NursingCenter%20eNews&utm_ campaign=1_NC%20eNews:%20 November%202014:%20Issue%201

International Family Nursing Association. (2013). *IFNA Position Paper on Pre-Licensure Family Nursing Education*. Retrieved from http:// internationalfamilynursing.org/wordpress/ wp-content/uploads/2015/07/FNE-.

International Family Nursing Association. (2015). *IFNA Position Paper on Generalist Competencies for Family Nursing Practice*. Retrieved from http:// internationalfamilynursing.org/wordpress/ wp-content/uploads/2015/07/GC-

Krumwiede, N., & Royle, C. (2011). Self-efficacy questionnaire. Unpublished instrument. School of Nursing, Minnesota State University, Mankato, MN.

Krumwiede, N., Royle, C., & Groteluschen, W. (2011). Knowledge acquisition questionnaire. Unpublished instrument. School of Nursing, Minnesota State University, Mankato, MN.

Krumwiede, N., Royle, C., & Moon, M. (2015). Family awareness and sensitivity tool. Unpublished instrument. School of Nursing, Minnesota State University, Mankato, MN.

Meiers, S. J., Eggenberger, S. K., & Krumwiede, N. K. (2016, March). *Testing and scoring of the family illness experience scale: Chronic illness*. Poster presentation at the 40th Annual Research Conference of the Midwest Nursing Research Society. Milwaukee, Wisconsin.

Price, C. A., Bush, K. R., & Price, S. J. (2017). *Families & change: Coping with stressful events and transitions* (5th ed.). Los Angeles, CA: Sage.

Sawin, K. J., & Harrigan, M. P. (1995). Measures of family functioning for research and practice. New York, NY: Springer Publishing Co.

Svavarsdottir, E. K., Sigurdardottir, A. O., Konradsdottir, E., Stefansdottir, A., Sveinbjarnardottir, E. K., Ketilsdottir, A., . . . Guðmundsdottir, H. (2015). The process of translating family nursing knowledge into clinical practice. *Journal of Nursing Scholarship, 47*(1), 5–15. doi: 10.1111/ jnu.12108

Wright, L. M., & Leahey, M. (2013). Nurses and families: A guide to family assessment and intervention (6th ed). Philadelphia, PA: F. A. Davis.

Young, P. K., Krumwiede, N. K., & Eggenberger, S. K. (2016, March). *Family nursing practice patterns of graduating baccalaureate nursing students*. Poster presentation at the 40th Annual Research Conference of the Midwest Nursing Research Society. Milwaukee, Wisconsin.

12

Thinking Like a Nurse: Optimizing Clinical Judgment and Reasoning Through the ACE.S Unfolding Cases

Colleen Royle, EdD, MSN, RN
MaryAnn McKenna Moon, MSN, APRN, ACNS-BC
Norma Krumwiede, EdD, MEd, MN, RN
Stacey Van Gelderen, DNP, RN
Kelly Krumwiede, PhD, RN, PHN
Walter Groteluschen, MS

OVERVIEW

A team of educators taught nursing students to think like a nurse (Tanner, 2006) using ACE.S Unfolding Cases to encourage improved understandings of complexities of care, geriatric syndromes and transition of care for older adults. Faculty trialed approaches to clinical simulations, and developed tools in order to determine the most effective method of optimizing knowledge based decision-making by students. These simulation cases address the essential knowledge domains and implement nursing actions appropriate for older adults.

DEVELOPMENT AND IMPLEMENTATION

The School of Nursing faculty at Minnesota State University, Mankato is committed to guiding nursing students in developing a practice based on innovative models of care. Integrating the Advancing Care Excellence for Seniors (ACE.S) Framework and Unfolding Case Studies assists undergraduate nursing students to gain new understandings of individualized aging processes, complexities in aging, and life transitions with aging family members. Students use a model of clinical judgment proposed by Tanner (2006) that includes four phases of noticing, interpreting, responding, and reflecting that occur when the ACE.S Unfolding Cases are used to teach gerontological nursing practice and concepts.

In 2012, the faculty attended the Innovations in Teaching: An ACE.S workshop in Lincoln, Nebraska and committed to integrate gerontologic nursing content throughout the curriculum using ACE.S (http://www.nln.org/professional-development-programs/teaching-resources/aging) and *Consult Geri* (https://consultgeri.org/) resources. The teaching-learning strategy of unfolding case studies (Reese, 2011) assists students to become safe, practical and competent nurses by attaching assessment and interventions plans to stories that unfold over time. This pedagogy embraces a constructivist learning framework (Peters, 2000), curricular scaffolding approach, and narrative pedagogy (Ironside, 2015). During the workshop, faculty learned to use a common language to examine and develop several core elements of this innovative approach to teaching: (a) the use of high-fidelity mannequins and standardized patients to teach geriatric nursing, (b) comparing oral debriefing and video-assisted debriefing in providing meaningful experience for students, and (c) intentionally incorporating family nursing actions and family as a recipient of care into each of the Unfolding Cases. After attending the ACE.S workshop, faculty met throughout the summer to strategically implement the NLN's ACE.S Unfolding Cases into existing curriculum.

All four of the ACE.S Unfolding Cases: Millie Larsen, Red Yoder, Henry Williams, and Julia Morales and Lucy Grey are implemented in a consistent manner throughout the curriculum. For example, when running Millie Larsen, simulation scenarios 1, 2, and 3 proceed consecutively within a 3- to 4-hour period so students can comprehend the transitions of care where most errors occur. Initially, each student was given a paper packet that included presimulation work developed from the NLN ACE.S Unfolding Case simulation scenarios 1, 2, and 3, and the Hartford Institute for Geriatric Nursing assessment tools for older adults. The prework section consisted of the monologue of the client and family describing their health and illness experience, the context, and evidence-based articles that clarify or support the simulation foci. Each simulation scenario included the simulation design template, learning objectives for faculty and students, protocols or algorithms used in the simulation, client's chart, family data and family concerns, and any additional monologue specific to that simulation. The Hartford tools required in the simulations, such as SPICES, Geriatric Depression Scale, and Confusion Assessment Method were available for students to review prior to the simulation (How to Try This Series, 2016).

Initially, faculty chose to have four of the students participate in the actual scenario and live stream the simulation to the remaining class of 36 students. Even though learning occurred, student satisfaction with the overall experience was extremely low due to their lack of engagement in the simulation. A second approach was implemented. The class was divided in half so more students could actively participate in a scenario; however, faculty satisfaction diminished with a lack of student engagement and limited student learning about care transitions. Therefore, the next approach of engaging small groups with an ideal number of 10 to12 students involved in each simulation case was adopted. Four different students participated in each of the three scenarios of the actual simulation and the remaining students observe in an adjacent room through a live feed audio/video system.

Simulation learning experiences with the ACE.S Unfolding Cases occur during students' clinical time. Each of the four Unfolding Cases is scheduled approximately every other week during the clinical rotation which allows faculty to build on prior learning in clinical settings and simulate real-world experiences. The four Unfolding Cases are given in this order: (a) Millie Larsen (individualized aging: communication, UTI, and delirium), (b) Red Yoder (complexity of care: teaching and threat of abuse), (c) Henry Williams (vulnerability during transitions: multiple care management issues), then (d) Julia Morales and Lucy Grey (individualized aging, complexity of care, and vulnerability during transitions). The faculty use all three scenarios of the Unfolding Cases sequentially over three hours. Structuring the learning with a sequential and intermingled approach to simulation enhanced students' understanding of the complexity of care, geriatric syndromes, and transition of care.

In order to further enhance student engagement, two tools were developed: (a) Peer Observation & Feedback Tool (Christian & Krumwiede, 2011; see Box 12.1) and (b) Clinical Judgment and Reasoning Tool (Krumwiede, 2011; see Box 12.2). Half of the student observers were

---

BOX 12.1

Peer Observation & Feedback Tool, ACE.S Simulation: Millie Larsen

Formative Feedback	Comments/ Student Feedback

Nursing Process:
How did the simulation experience progress?
Did the nurse ask appropriate questions of the client and family?
Is there any information you feel you still need that the team didn't collect?
Would it have been helpful to explore obtaining further information from the family member?

Critical Thinking:
Did the team address your concerns for the client?
Did the team address your concerns for the family?
Did the team identify the cause of your concern?

Communication:
Did the team acknowledge the family experience?
Did the team utilize SBAR communication?
Did the team invite the family into the experience?

Therapeutic Intervention:
Did the team intervene appropriately?
Did the team acknowledge the client's response to interventions?
Did the team therapeutically respond to families cues?

Role Development:
Who was the leader?
Who emerged as the leader?
Did you observe delegation? Explain

Coordinating Care:
How did the team work together?
Did the team communicate effectively?
Did the team understand each other's role in caring for the client?
Did the team collaborate in caring for the family?

What went well with this simulation?

What could have been done differently?

Copyright © Minnesota State University, Mankato, School of Nursing Faculty, 2016.

BOX 12.2

Clinical Judgment and Reasoning Tool, ACE.S Simulation: Millie Larsen

Noticing
1. What is the primary concern that you have for Millie's family?
2. What is the primary concern that you have for Millie?
3. What is your primary concern for Snuggles?
4. What nursing knowledge or evidence assists you with Millie's case?

Interpreting (Prioritizing Data)
1. As the nurse, which of the signs and symptoms discovered above is of greatest concern to you?
2. Which findings require your immediate attention?

Responding
1. What steps would you take to address the priority concerns in Millie Larsen's case?
2. How would you go about implementing your actions without alarming the patient or family?

Reflecting
1. What insight does this exercise give you into caring for the family of a frail elder?
2. What insight does this exercise give you into caring for the individual with stress incontinence, UTI and confusion?
3. What insight does this exercise give you into caring for the geriatric population?

These questions were developed from Tanner's Clinical Judgment Model (2006).
Copyright © Minnesota State University, Mankato, School of Nursing Faculty, 2016.

given the Peer Observation & Feedback Tool that focuses on nursing process, critical thinking, communication, therapeutic intervention, role development, and coordinating care to identify positive learning with simulation and those areas needing improvement. The other half of the student observers were given the Clinical Judgment and Reasoning Tool that includes specific questions regarding the scenario that address the four phases of noticing, interpreting, responding, and reflecting (Tanner, 2006).

Because reflections from the students who assumed the roles of nurses or family members is central to the learning experience, the Reflective Thinking Tool (Krumwiede & Royle, 2012; see Box 12.3) was administered to the students in the scenario. The tool developed from Carper's Fundamental Patterns of Knowing for nursing (1978) asks questions pertaining to each of the patterns of knowing and prompts the student to engage in the reflective process of nursing practice. The Family Awareness and Sensitivity Tool (Krumwiede, Royle, & Moon, 2015; see Box 11.2 in Chapter 11) focuses on the experience of the family member. These tools are completed at the end of the scenario by the four students with direct involvement in the simulation.

EVALUATION

During fall semester 2012, one of the NLN ACE.S project team members, made a site visit to observe the Henry Williams Unfolding Case and offered the following feedback:

BOX 12.3

Reflective Thinking Tool, ACE.S Simulation: Millie Larsen

Empirical—What knowledge informed your nursing actions?
Aesthetic—What particular issues seem significant to pay attention to?
Personal—What factors influenced the way you felt, thought, or responded?
Ethical—To what extent did you act for the best and remain in tune with your values?
Reflection—How might you respond more effectively given this situation again?
Family & Societal—How did you address the needs of the family?

These questions were developed from Carper's *Fundamental Patterns of Knowing for Nursing* (1978). Copyright © Minnesota State University, Mankato, School of Nursing Faculty, 2016.

(a) offering all three scenarios in one day was beneficial for students to identify potential gaps or errors during times of transition; (b) faculty efforts to develop tools to measure student self-efficacy, knowledge acquisition, and satisfaction were encouraging; and (c) the Peer Observation & Feedback Tool, the Clinical Judgment and Reasoning Tool, the Reflective Thinking Tool, and the Family Awareness and Sensitivity Tool fostered a sense of higher order thinking, and deeper significant learning through reflective nursing practice. One student upon completion of the Julia Morales and Lucy Grey simulation, reflected on the experience:

> *I think I kind of failed her…I would pay more attention to what the patient is actually saying and not worry so much about my objectives. I also think I wasn't as confident as I wanted to be throughout the scenario. I often felt unsure and was afraid to engage with a same sex couple.*

Another student reflected on the Henry William's Unfolding Case, that during simulation students must *"prepare very well, act like a real nurse and be attentive to the needs of the patient and the family. Prioritize care and communicate with patient and family throughout."*

Faculty believe that the success experienced with the use of the ACE.S Unfolding Cases during simulation experiences is due to the NLN's vision to transform geriatric nursing practice by re-conceptualizing nursing education. This approach to learning supports how nurses are prepared-for and engaged-in the care of older adults and their families while maintaining the NLN's core values of caring, integrity, diversity, and excellence. Thus, faculty continue to integrate the NLN ACE.S Framework to teach nursing students how to provide competent, individualized care for older adults. For us, the real winners are the older adults and their families and communities who will benefit from nurses prepared to address the ACE.S Essential Knowledge Domains (individualized aging, complexity of care, or vulnerability during transitions), geriatric syndromes (delirium, falls, incontinence, eating or feeding problems, sleep problems, or skin issues) and incorporate the ACE.S Essential Nursing Actions (assess functions and expectations, coordinate and manage care, use evolving knowledge, or situational decisions).

By examining the students' performance and knowledge acquisition, faculty determined that using the ACE.S Unfolding Cases was an effective teaching strategy. This innovative and deliberative approach to simulations encourages students to a thinking process with their nursing practice. While thinking like a nurse, students were able to model and role model clinical judgment and reasoning and offer suggestions on how to improve decision-making when their thinking became faulty. The reflection and evaluation processes encourage students to continue acquiring ongoing assessment and evaluation thinking skills.

As faculty reflect on what has been accomplished since instituting the NLN ACE.S simulation program at our university, the following questions have emerged:

1. How do we measure knowledge transfer and knowledge use in the moment?
2. How could we use the NLN ACE.S Framework to evaluate students in practice?
3. How do we measure the impact of student learning on the quality-of-care outcomes (financial strain, medication errors, and changes in functionality) and the quality-of-care challenges (communication, planning, coordination of care, addressing frailty, and family-focused and caregiver education)?

Faculty are currently engaged in research and education teams to address each of these questions.

References

Carper, B. A. (1978). Fundamental patterns of knowing in nursing, *Advances in Nursing Science, 1*(1), 13–24.

Christian, A., & Krumwiede, N. (2011). Peer observation & feedback tool. Unpublished instrument. School of Nursing, Minnesota State University, Mankato, MN.

How to Try This Series. (2016). Lippincott Learning Center. Retrieved from http://www.nursingcenter.com/static?pageid=730390&utm_source=WhatCountsEmail&utm_medium=NursingCenter%20eNews&utm_campaign=1_NC%20eNews:%20November%202014:%20Issue%201

Ironside, P. (2015). Narrative pedagogy: Transforming nursing education through 15 years of research in nursing education. *Nursing Education Perspectives, 36*(2), 83–88.

Krumwiede, N. (2011). Clinical judgment and reasoning tool. Unpublished instrument.

School of Nursing, Minnesota State University, Mankato, MN.

Krumwiede, N., & Royle, C. (2012). Reflective thinking tool. Unpublished instrument. School of Nursing, Minnesota State University, Mankato, MN.

Krumwiede, N., Royle, C., & Moon, M. (2015). Family awareness and sensitivity tool. Unpublished instrument. School of Nursing, Minnesota State University, Mankato, MN.

Peters, M. (2000). Does constructivist epistemology have a place in nursing education? *Journal of Nursing Education, 39*(4), 166–172.

Reese, C. (2011). Unfolding case studies. *Journal of Continuing Education in Nursing, 42*(8), 344–45.

Tanner, C. A. (2006). Thinking like a nurse: A research-based model of clinical judgment in nursing. *Journal of Nursing Education, 45*(6), 204–211.

13

A One-Day Geriatric Seminar Using ACE.S Resources

Vivienne Friday, EdD, RN

OVERVIEW

The population age 65 and over increased from 35.9 million in 2003 to 44.7 million in 2013 (a 24.7 percent increase) and is projected to more than double to 98 million by 2060. By 2040, there will be about 82.3 million older persons, over twice their number in 2000 (U.S. Department of Health and Human Services, 2014).

These statistics, as well as statistics about chronic illness and associated difficulties with activities of daily living (ADLs) and instrumental activities of daily living (IADLs), indicate the need for a more robust infusion of geriatric content in the nursing curriculum of a Midwestern community college. Ninety-seven percent of institutionalized Medicare beneficiaries have difficulty with one or more ADLs, and 83 percent have difficulty with three or more IADLs. (ADLs include bathing, dressing, eating, and mobility around the house. IADLs include shopping, preparing meals, using the telephone, and taking medications.) With increases in the number of chronic illnesses among older adults, functional disabilities intensify (U.S. Census Bureau, 2014).

A curriculum redesign, piloted by this author, resulted in several focused learning activities, including a one-day geriatric seminar offered to senior nursing students. The seminar is designed so that students, working in groups, research, review, and present sessions to peers, focusing on issues that impact quality of care for older adults. Students care for older adults in a wide variety of clinical settings throughout the program of learning; the seminar was designed to provide additional course work related to the care of older adults and their caregivers.

DEVELOPMENT AND IMPLEMENTATION

The seminar was based on the NLN ACE.S teaching strategy *Student-Led Geriatric Nursing Conference: Evidence in Practice* (NLN, 2016). Components of the ACE.S framework were incorporated into the seminar to provide focus for the experience. Students addressed the area of individualized aging by conducting interviews with older adults in the community or by participating in discussions about a movie that addresses sexuality and the older adult. Students studied complexity of care and vulnerability during transitions by participating in the ACE.S Henry and Ertha Williams Unfolding Case study (Cleary, 2016).

Students were placed in groups of five and given three assignments. One assignment required them to research key issues relevant to older adults. Suggestions included: advance directives, re-admission into hospitals within 30 days, caregiver strain, and cultural beliefs that impact treatment and medication compliance. For the second assignment, students completed an assessment of an older adult using the SPICES tool, followed by a focused assessment based on initial assessment findings. The third assignment involved an interview of an older adult living in the community, including the identification of environmental needs and available resources. Many students chose to interview a family member for this assignment.

Group assignments were distributed four weeks prior to the seminar. Each group planned a 30–45 minute presentation to highlight and discuss with peers findings from their interviews and research. Presentations were done during the first half of the day. During the second half of the day, students participated in the ACE.S Unfolding Case of Henry and Ertha Williams, during which students remained in their assigned groups and formulated their own ending of the story.

The idea of finishing the story comes from a learning tool that accompanies each unfolding case. Students are asked to relate how they see Henry or Ertha about three months after their last encounter with them. How have they progressed? What issues have arisen for them? This assignment, whether accomplished in a log or group discussion, provides faculty with insight into what students have learned from the unfolding case. Finally, the seminar ended with a movie that focused on sexuality and the older adult. The movie of choice was "Grumpier Old Men."

EVALUATION

Using a teacher-designed feedback evaluation form at the end of the seminar, more than 90 percent of the students identified the seminar as extremely useful and informative or informative. Students also submitted a reflective journal one week after the seminar. The following student comments reveal an appreciation for the complexity of changes experienced by older adults and the need to more fully respond to the unique needs of older adults during transitions in order to provide individualized care.

> *"During this experience it really made me think about the booming elderly population and how much they really need help to adjust into the world. We need more people who are willing to help and are patient in providing care."*
>
> *"I completed the SPICES assessment and then a focused assessment on my grandmother. I realized that my grandma was dealing with many issues that other elderly people have. She is losing her independence. She is no longer allowed to drive, so she has to rely on others to take her places. When I was recently in the hospital, she had to wait till my mother could come pick her up. I could understand how this would become frustrating. She also doesn't get to see her friends as often as she used to. When she had her license, she would go get lunch with her friends almost every day. Now, most of the family members that drive her to visit her friends work during the day. She has to wait alone all day until people get off work and can take her places.*
>
> *Loneliness is a major worry for the elderly. My grandmother had never lived alone in her entire life. She lived with her parents and then her husband. Now that her husband is gone, she has no one to talk to 24 hours a day and take care of. Many elderly people find this*

difficult and suffer depression. I had no idea she was so sad and I am sure this is the case in many other families. Thankfully, my grandmother is getting help; but what about the elderly who are too embarrassed to get help or who think it is a normal aging process?"

"I feel the time spent on case studies (Henry and Ertha) and meeting with one another to discuss the case studies was very beneficial."

"First I strongly dislike doing case studies but this one I believe was beneficial. Cultural competence is something I had never heard of before. It was interesting because even when discussing the case studies we all had different viewpoints. This was able to shine some light on how every individual is different, and how ethical decision-making is not black and white".

References

Cleary, J. (2016). Henry and Ertha Williams [ACE.S Unfolding Cases]. Retrieved from http://www.nln.org/professional-development-programs/teaching-resources/aging/ace-s/unfolding-cases/henry-and-ertha-williams

The National League for Nursing (NLN). (2016). *Student-led geriatric nursing conference: Evidence in practice* [ACE.S Teaching Strategy]. Retrieved from http://www.nln.org/professional-development-programs/teaching-resources/aging/ace-s/teaching-strategies/aces-knowledge-domains/complexity-of-care/student-led-geriatric-nursing-conference-evidence-in-practice

U.S. Census Bureau (2014). *American community survey*. Retrieved from https://www.census.gov/programs-surveys/acs/

U.S. Department of Health and Human Services Administration on Aging. (2015). A profile of older Americans: 2015. Retrieved from http://www.aoa.acl.gov/aging_statistics/profile/2014/docs/2014-Profile.pdf

14

Helping Students Process a Simulated Death Experience: Integration of an NLN ACE.S Evolving Case Study and the ELNEC Curriculum

Judith A. Kopka, MSN, RN, CNE
Ann P. Aschenbrenner, PhD, RN, CNE
Mary B. Reynolds, MSN/ED, RN

ABSTRACT

The nursing literature supports the need for end-of-life (EOL) education, but the ability to provide quality clinical experience in this area is limited by the availability of patients and nursing instructors' and preceptors' comfort and expertise in teaching EOL care. Clinical simulation allows faculty to provide the same quality EOL experience to all students. This chapter discusses an effective teaching strategy integrating End-of-Life Nursing Education Consortium core content with National League for Nursing ACE.S unfolding case studies, clinical simulation, and social media.

OVERVIEW

The need for end-of-life (EOL) care in the nursing curriculum has been well documented, but standard teaching strategies are often inadequate. This article describes an effective teaching strategy for pre-licensure nursing students that integrates the End-of-Life Nursing Education Consortium (ELNEC) core curriculum, the National League for Nursing (NLN) Advancing Care Excellence for Seniors (ACE.S) Unfolding Case studies, clinical simulation, and social media, specifically Facebook. The focus was on helping students process a patient death and gain confidence and skills when interacting with a dying patient and the patient's family. This fourfold teaching strategy for EOL care proved to be efficient, engaging for faculty and students, and successful in improving students' skills in this critically important area.

The simulation took place as part of a three-credit didactic gerontology course for senior nursing students. Preparation for the simulation began with the ELNEC curriculum known as ELNEC-Core (American Association of Colleges of Nursing [AACN], 2000), introduced concurrently with the NLN ACE.S Unfolding Case study on Julia Morales and Lucy Grey (Cato, 2012; NLN, n.d.). Both were used throughout the course in large and small groups. Prior to the simulation, students watched the video "Evan Mayday's Good Death" (www.med.umich.edu/nursing/EndOfLife/mayday.htm) and completed an individual reflection. Faculty members led student discussion about the film.

To enhance realism, a Facebook page was developed for Julia, the ACE.S character. Students could "friend" or email Julia, and faculty responded as Julia. The course culminated in a simulated death experience for groups of 10 students. The teaching strategies are summarized in Table 14.1.

TABLE 14.1

Teaching Strategies for End-of-Life Simulation

Teaching Strategies	Implementation
The simulation was conducted during the final class of the semester as part of a 3-credit didactic gerontology course. Preparation included class and online modules on the ELNEC core curriculum.	Introduce the Julia Morales and Lucy Grey ACE.S Unfolding Case study throughout the ELNEC core curriculum. ELNEC topics (pain management, caregiving, and symptom management) were integrated throughout the last five weeks of the course, with Julia and her caregiver Lucy and son Neil as patient and family during small group work and discussion activities.
Use of Social Media	Develop a realistic Facebook page for Julia with pictures of Julia and Lucy, their travels and family, and "Likes," such as favorite sports teams. Students are required to either "friend" Julia and post a comment on her wall or send her an email. Faculty respond as Julia.
Simulation	A high-fidelity manikin is dressed and placed in a small room decorated to look like a home environment. The manikin is programmed to display common signs of impending death, including Cheyne-Stokes respirations with lengthening intervals of apnea progressing to death. Faculty enact a loosely scripted role-play of the interaction involving the hospice nurse, Julia's son Neil, and partner Lucy based on the ACE.S simulation template. After approximately 10 minutes, Julia dies, and the hospice nurse offers to make necessary calls and provides sympathy, reassurance, and hugs to the grieving family.
Evaluation	Faculty conduct a 20-minute focus group for debriefing after the simulation, encouraging students to share their responses and process feelings that arose during the simulation. A written questionnaire incorporating debriefing questions from the ACE.S case study is distributed. Faculty added questions on students' reactions to the death. Students complete this anonymously, allowing them to provide feedback they may not feel comfortable sharing in a group.

EDUCATIONAL PREPARATION

Dying is an intrinsic part of life, and nursing curricula need enriched didactic and clinical content on EOL care (Allchin, 2006). Classes on the end of life for baccalaureate students generally stir feelings of fear and hesitancy (Allchin). White and Coyne (2011) found that many students reported having only two hours or less of EOL education in the preceding two years.

According to the Institute of Medicine (2008), the number of older adults in the United States will nearly double by 2030, leading to a need for nurses who are competent and comfortable in providing quality EOL care. The AACN published competencies for EOL care for older adults in 2010. ELNEC offers modules on pain and symptom management, ethics, communication, and other key EOL issues (AACN, 2000).

Simulation can be an effective means of preparing students to address EOL issues effectively and compassionately. A key to providing effective education through simulation and enhancing clinical reasoning is the realism and complexity of the scenario. The NLN ACE.S initiative (n.d.) is designed to improve care of older adults by providing curriculum resources, unfolding case studies, and teaching strategies. ACE.S Unfolding Cases are evidence-based and include first-person monologues and simulation templates for classroom, clinical, and skills lab activities; they can be modified to meet individual course and curriculum needs.

The Unfolding Case used as the basis for this simulation involved Julia Morales, age 65, her son Neil, and her partner of 25 years, Lucy Grey. The three scenarios offered by ACE.S begin with Julia's story and her current battle with lung cancer, continue to her death, and conclude with her grieving partner, Lucy, in the emergency department.

This class used the second scenario, which was adapted to be observational rather than interactive, with faculty conducting the role-play; debriefing conducted by faculty followed immediately after the simulation. The case study was expanded to incorporate core ELNEC curricula, and both Julia and Lucy were considered patients throughout the final five weeks of the course. Faculty-led discussions focused on ethics from the perspective of Julia's decision to stop treatment, and quality of life and caregiver burden as Lucy took on more of Julia's care. Students were very familiar with Julia and Lucy by the time of Julia's death. The Facebook page was used to enhance the reality of the characters. (See Table 14.1.)

SUMMARY AND EVALUATION

Students responded positively to the Facebook page, as social media are an integral part of their daily activity. Schmitt, Sims-Giddens, and Booth (2012) support the use of social media as a means to help students gain in understanding and skill. In this case, Facebook was used to enhance empathy, a quality vital for caring for dying patients and their families. Students shared that they felt they actually knew Julia and Lucy, which made Julia's death real to them. At first, Julia received numerous Facebook "friend" requests from across the country, but by changing the Facebook settings, limiting access to students, and identifying Julia as a "fictional person," this problem was resolved.

The use of the ACE.S case study facilitated the implementation of the simulation. Teaching resources provided for faculty enhanced the realism and quality of the scenarios; these included the evaluation tool provided with the ACE.S unfolding case studies as well as case study content and simulation templates and scripts. Faculty added questions to the debriefing specific to students' feelings about EOL issues and their perceived ability to address these issues after the simulation.

Feedback from students supported the effectiveness of this teaching strategy in increasing their comfort with the dying process and helping them communicate with patients and their families. Comments on the death included: "Felt sad but peaceful that it was such a nice environment for her to die in" and "I felt emotional and connected to the experience." Feedback on the simulation as a learning activity included: "Beneficial. I think I will remember this when I come across it in my nursing career." One student stated: "Helped me know what to say to patient and family at EOL. Support is so important to help patient and family have a good death experience." Another described it as the "best learning experience I ever had."

References

Allchin, L. (2006). Caring for the dying: Nursing student perspectives. *Journal of Hospice and Palliative Care, 8*(2), 112–117.

American Association of Colleges of Nursing. (2000). *ELNEC-Core.* Retrieved from www.aacn.nche.edu/elnec/about/elnec-core

American Association of Colleges of Nursing. (2010). *Recommended baccalaureate competencies and curricular guidelines for the nursing care of older adults*. Retrieved from www.aacn.nche.edu/geriatric-nursing/AACN_Gerocompetencies.pdf

Cato, M. L. (2012). Julia Morales and Lucy Grey [ACE.S Unfolding Cases]. Retrieved from www.nln.org/professional-development-programs/teaching-resources/aging/unfolding-cases/julia-morales-and-lucy-grey

Institute of Medicine. (2008). *Retooling for an aging America: Building the health care workforce.* Washington, DC: National Academies Press.

National League for Nursing. (n.d.). NLN Center for Excellence in the Care of Vulnerable Populations. Retrieved from www.nln.org/centers-for-nursing-education/nln-center-for-excellence-in-the-care-of-vulnerable-populations

Schmitt, T., Sims-Giddens, S., & Booth, R. (2012). Social media use in nursing education. *Online Journal of Issues in Nursing, 17*(3), Manuscript 2. doi:10.3912/OJIN.Vol17No03Man02

White, K. R., & Coyne, P. J. (2011). Nurses' perception of educational gaps in delivering end-of-life care. *Oncology Nurse Forum, 38*(6), 711–717.